CONTENTS

HEADWAY LIFEGUIDES

MASSAGE

Denise Brown

*To my dear husband Garry for his patience and understanding and
my two water babies, Chloë and Thomas*

The publishers would like to thank the following: for giving permission
to reproduce copyright photographic material in this book, Zefa Picture
Library, p. 6, Foto Scala, Florence, p. 7; Roddy Paine for all
commissioned photographs; Jennie Brown for the anatomical drawings
and Helen Reed for the plant drawings.

British Library Cataloguing in Publication Data

Brown, Denise
  Massage – (Headway Lifeguides Series)
  I. Title II Series
  615.8

  ISBN 0–340–55949–7

First published 1993

Typeset by Wearset, Boldon, Tyne and Wear
Printed in Great Britain for the educational publishing division of Hodder & Stoughton Ltd, Mill
Road, Dunton Green, Sevenoaks, Kent by Thomson Litho Ltd

INTRODUCTION

Our instinctive need for touch

To touch and to be touched is a fundamental instinctive need in all of us whatever our age. Human life itself is the result of a man and woman joining together and, as the sperm and ovum unite, new life develops from their contact. The first sense that the embryo develops is that of the sense of touch. Rocked and nourished in the mother's womb the unborn child is wrapped in a constant embrace. This close bond with the mother is the basis for the human need for touch and it is this closeness and warmth of the womb that we seek throughout our life.

Even during the process of labour and birth the powerful uterine contractions which squeeze and push us along the birth canal continue this massage effect. Evidence seems to indicate that babies who do not experience a 'normal' delivery may experience some developmental disadvantages due to the lack of the touching sensations of birth. Such infants require frequent amounts of touching and massage. It is of the utmost importance that close physical contact between mother and baby be maintained directly after the birth. Close bonding appears to have a positive effect on weight gain and reduces infections during the first years of life.

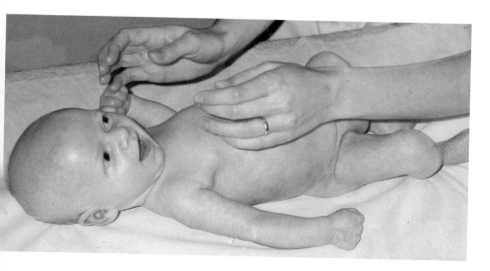

Touching has an enormous impact on the formation of the personality and on our ability to participate and respond in loving relationships later on in life. Children who grow up in families where there is deprivation of touch are generally less healthy, less able to withstand pain and infection, less confident and less happy. Loving and secure personalities emerge from families where there is an abundance of touch.

Touch means security and comfort. Massage is merely an extended form of touch. To massage is an instinctive medicine which we all have at our command. As a child we instinctively attempt to massage away aches and pains and as an adult we may stroke the brow and shoulders of a weary and distressed friend. We *all* have the power in our hands to alleviate the everyday tensions, aches and pains using just a few simple massage techniques as described in this book.

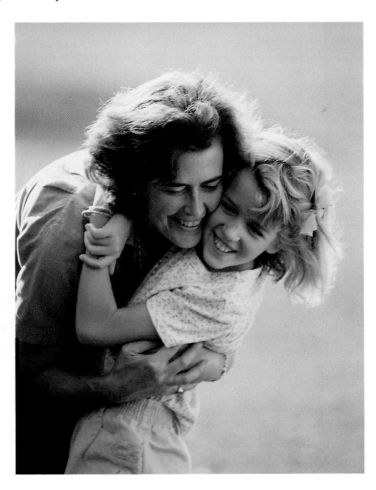

A brief history of massage

The healing art of massage, probably derived from the French word *masser*, is undoubtedly the oldest form of medical treatment known to humanity. It was practised by the Chinese three thousand years before the birth of Christ to prevent, soothe and heal pain. Ancient documents testify to the fact that massage therapy was practised amongst the Greeks and Romans. Hippocrates, the 'Father of Medicine', is renowned for his statement in the fifth century BC that 'rubbing can bind a joint which is too loose, and loosen a joint that is too rigid'. In ancient Rome Julius Caesar had daily massage to treat his neuralgia and the Roman writer Pliny was regularly massaged to alleviate his asthma.

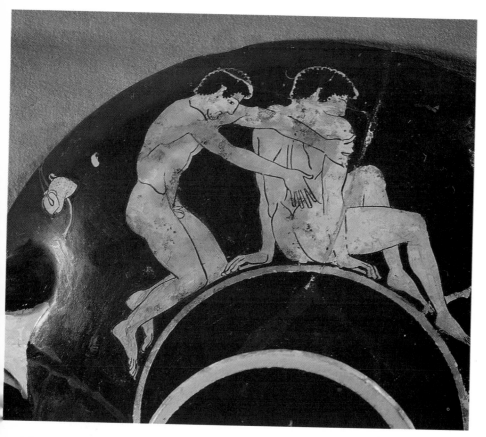

After the decline of the Roman Empire there is little reference to massage and medicine until the Middle Ages when interest in the art of massage was regenerated. The French physician Ambrose Paré advocated the use of massage for stiff and injured joints and established its credibility within the medical profession. Professor Peter Henry Ling established a school of massage in Stockholm. Massage grew in popularity and Ling's techniques became known as 'Swedish massage'.

At the present time there is a rapidly growing demand for all forms of natural therapy. The preventative and therapeutic art of massage is now developing and flourishing and gaining recognition all over the world. Many hundreds of thousands of people are now enjoying the remarkable benefits that it can offer. Even in orthodox medicine, massage is becoming increasingly accepted as a therapy. Many nurses, aware of the value of touch, are now studying the art of massage at my college with the aim of incorporating it into their work. Massage plays an important role in the control of pain brought about by the release of endorphins and is employed in some enlightened maternity wards together with essential oils to ease the discomforts of labour and to promote calmness in the mother-to-be. In geriatric wards it reduces the need for drugs in cases of insomnia and constipation and carries no risk of side effects. In hospices the healing language of touch helps to alleviate not only physical problems but also engenders a feeling of peace and serenity allowing the sick and dying to retain their dignity. All forms of orthodox medicine may be complemented by the power of the healing hands for which there is no substitute.

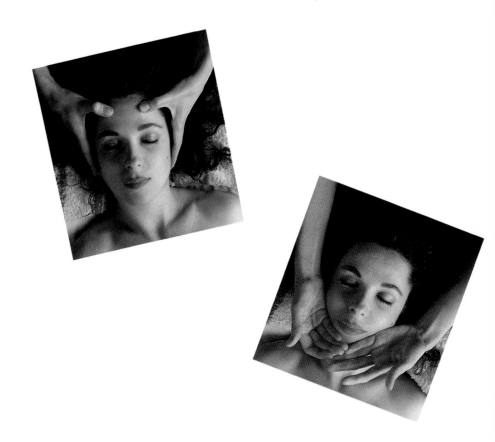

The value of massage

Massage is essential to the promotion and maintenance of good health. It has enormous therapeutic effects, both physiological and psychological, on all the systems of the body. The nervous system will benefit because the stresses and strains of modern day living may be considerably alleviated and all types of headaches may be relieved. Neck, shoulder and back pain will be reduced and the discomforts of arthritis and rheumatism suffered by so many can be relieved. The lymphatic system is stimulated, thereby assisting the elimination of toxins and poisons, cleansing and purifying our systems more efficiently. The circulatory and immune systems are activated. Digestion is improved and constipation and bowel problems subside. The respiratory system benefits as breathing and bronchial disorders are improved.

In short, massage is capable of inducing an excellent state of well-being and harmony. What is more, the benefits of massage are not only felt by the receiver but also by the masseur. Whilst giving a treatment we experience a total sense of relaxation as we immerse ourselves and on completion we feel revived, revitalised and full of energy!

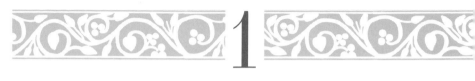

1

SETTING THE SCENE

Creating the right atmosphere

It is extremely important to pay particular attention to the environment in which the massage is to be performed if maximum benefit is to be derived from the treatment. Careful preparation and the right setting will make a good massage even better! The environment should be arranged so that both giver and receiver feel immediately relaxed just by being there. Always ensure that all towels, cushions and oils are on hand so as not to lose contact and thus break the flow of the massage.

Pay careful attention to the following:

Solitude and quiet
These are vital. Ensure that you choose a time when you will not be disturbed. Intrusions and distractions are extremely disconcerting, breaking your concentration and destroying the flow of your massage movements. Take the telephone off the hook and tell your friends and family not to enter the treatment room. You may decide to choose some soothing background music although this is a matter of personal preference. Some will prefer silence.

Cleanliness
This is essential too. Always wash your hands before the treatment as any stickiness will be instantly obvious to the receiver. Make sure that fingernails are short – trim them as far down as possible. Do not wear any jewellery on the hands.

Warmth
The room should be draught-free and very warm yet well ventilated. Nothing will destroy a massage more quickly than physical coldness. It is impossible to relax when you feel cold. The room in which you give the massage should be heated prior to the treatment and, as the body temperature will drop, ensure that spare towels and blankets are at your disposal. All areas should be kept covered other than the part on which you are working. Warm your hands if they feel cold.

Lighting
Soft and subdued lighting will create the ideal atmosphere. Bright lights falling on the receiver's face will hardly induce relaxation and will cause tension around the eyes. Candlelight provides the perfect setting or you may wish to use a tinted bulb. Choose from pale pink, blue, green, peach or lavender.

Colour

The most therapeutic colours to have in the room are pastel shades – pale pink, blue, green or peach decor and towels are perfect for the occasion. Colours such as red will tend to create unwanted emotions like anger and restlessness.

Clothes

Wear comfortable and loose-fitting clothes as you need to move around easily and the room in which you will be working will be very warm. White is the best colour to wear when giving a massage since it will reflect any negativity which is released from the individual being treated.

Wear flat shoes or, even better, go barefoot. The receiver should undress down to whatever level they feel comfortable with. Suggest they undress down to at least their underwear. Point out that any areas which are not being worked on will be covered up as this will create a sense of security and trust.

Finishing touches

Use some fresh flowers to add a pleasant aroma to the atmosphere or even burn some incense or essential oils prior to the treatment. Crystals may also enhance the environment.

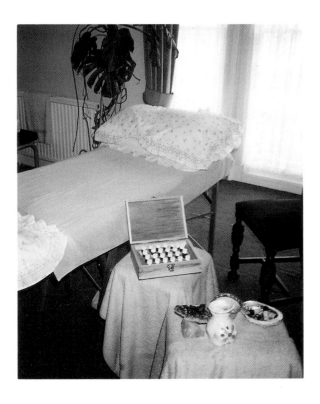

Equipment

Massage surface

You may work on the floor using a firm yet well padded surface. This will allow you to give a massage wherever you desire. Place a large, thick piece of foam or two or three blankets or a thick duvet on the floor. Use plenty of cushions during the massage. When the receiver is lying on the back, place

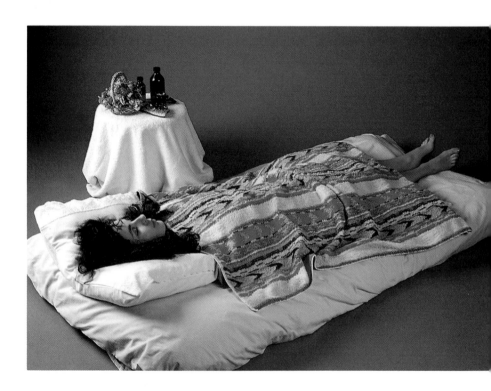

one under the head and one under the knees to take the pressure off the lower back.

When the receiver is lying on the front, place a cushion under the feet, one under the head and shoulders and perhaps one under the abdomen if desired.

Ensure that you have something to kneel on to avoid sore knees. If you are unfortunate enough to be a back sufferer or have knee problems it may be a good idea to invest in a portable couch. It is far less tiring and makes the body readily accessible. You could try improvising by using the kitchen table if the height is comfortable for you. **Do not** use a bed as most are far too soft and are such an awkward height that you will need a massage yourself when you finish! Most mattresses are too soft for massage purposes as any pressure applied is absorbed by the mattress.

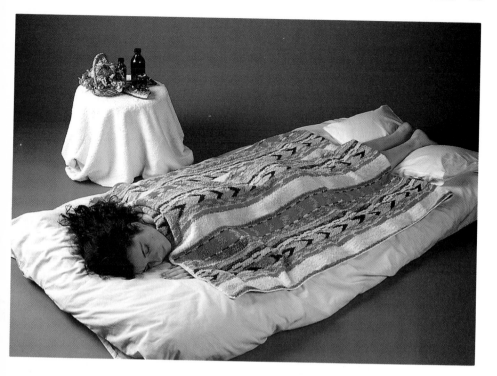

Oils

It is my opinion that the only really effective way to massage is with oil. This enables the hands to glide smoothly over the skin and the movements to flow freely. Some prefer to use talcum powder as a medium but I personally find it very restrictive and feel that it is unpleasant for both giver and receiver to inhale the powder.

Choose any good quality (cold-pressed, unrefined, additive-free) vegetable oil such as sweet almond, grapeseed, sunflower, safflower or soyabean. I do not recommend the use of mineral oil, such as baby oil, due to its low penetration power. Vegetable oil is easily absorbed and nourishing whereas mineral oil tends to clog the pores. You may decide to add a few drops of essential oil to enhance the treatment (see Chapter 4 on Aromatherapy).

Always keep the oil within easy reach during the treatment. Do not use too much oil as you will be unable to make proper contact and the receiver will feel most uncomfortable and sticky. A complete treatment actually requires very little oil – just a couple of tablespoons. If you wish, the oil may be warmed a little prior to the massage. **Never** pour oil directly onto the body. Pour about half a teaspoon onto the palm of one hand and then rub your hands together to warm the oil slightly before applying it. When you require more lubricant keep one hand in contact with the body. Breaking contact destroys the continuity of the massage and creates a feeling of insecurity.

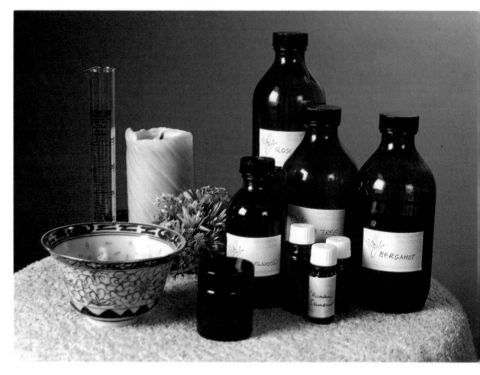

Your attitude and state of mind

Posture

Whether you are working on the floor or at a table, keep your back relaxed yet straight throughout the massage. Remember that it should be as relaxing to give a massage as it is to receive one. With practice you will learn to avoid tensing the muscles so that the healing energy can flow freely through your hands and body.

Attunement

Your state of mind when giving a massage is vital. The quality and success of a treatment depends upon having a calm state of mind. Do not attempt to give a massage when you are feeling angry, moody, depressed or unwell. Your negativity will be transmitted. Your complete attention must be devoted to the receiver. If you are worrying about your own problems and your mind is drifting then this will be communicated immediately.

Spend time consciously relaxing yourself prior to the treatment and, most importantly, be guided by your own intuition. Take a few deep breaths before the massage allowing all tension and anxiety to flow out of your body. Breathe in peace and breathe out love. Tune in to the person you are massaging. It may help to work with the eyes closed. Give yourself unselfishly to the massage.

Contraindications

Observe the following contraindications at all times:

High temperatures/fevers
The body is already fighting off toxins as indicated by the rise in temperature. A massage would release even more unwelcome toxins into the system.

Infectious skin conditions
These include ringworm, scabies and impetigo – you do not want to spread the condition or transfer it to yourself. Conditions such as acne, psoriasis and eczema are not infectious and may improve with the use of essential oils such as lavender. (Refer to my book on *Aromatherapy* in this series for information on specific skin conditions.)

Thrombo-phlebitis and other similar conditions
Phlebitis is inflammation of a vein. The skin near the inflamed vein is red, very hot and swollen. Considerable pain and tenderness to the touch are experienced along the vein. If a clot (thrombus) forms in the vein, massage is contraindicated since the clot could move, resulting in a fatality!

Advanced varicose veins
You risk the danger here of causing further inflammation and great pain.

Very recent scars or operations
Beware of recent scars and open wounds. Old scar tissue can be massaged.

Abdomen during pregnancy
Although massage is extremely beneficial, during pregnancy only very light massage should be applied to the abdominal area and lower back.

Lumps
These may be innocent but it is wise to have them investigated by a doctor.

2

BASIC STROKES

Massage *can* be simple! Even though there is a wide variety of different massage movements, most techniques are merely a variation on the strokes explained below. With the aid of these basic movements a complete body massage may be performed. As you develop and gain confidence you will invent your own strokes to build up an extensive repertoire.

Effleurage (stroking)

Description

Effleurage or stroking is one of the principal movements of massage which may be performed on any area of the body. It signals the beginning and the end of a massage both preceding and succeeding all other strokes and facilitating the flow from one movement to the next. The palms of both hands are used as you glide over the surface of the skin moulding your hands to the contours of the body. The receiver experiences one continuous movement as you apply firm, rhythmic pressure on the upward stroke yet glide downwards to your starting point with a featherlight touch. Close your eyes as you effleurage to accentuate and heighten your sensitivity and sense of touch.

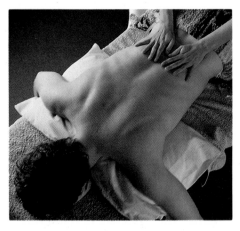 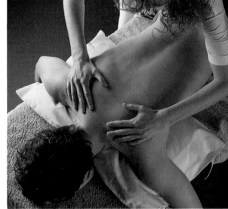

Benefits

The receiver experiences an immediate sense of well-being and relaxation. A relationship of trust is established between the two of you as your hands become accustomed to the receiver's body. Effleurage, when performed slowly, is particularly beneficial for soothing the nerves. Stress and strain may be relieved, tension headaches dispelled and patterns of insomnia broken. Brisk effleurage can be used to enliven, revive and stimulate. The tissues will warm up as you stroke the body, improving the circulation and increasing the flow of lymph to aid the elimination of waste and poisonous substances.

Errors to avoid

1 Do not lose contact with the receiver (loss of contact means loss of confidence).

2 Relax the hands and flow, avoiding any jerky or sudden movements (jerky movements create nervousness and irritation).

3 Use the whole hand and not just the fingertips (you can cover a much wider area).

4 *No* pressure whatsoever on the downward stroke (massage is always performed towards the heart).

Remember: if in doubt, effleurage! everyone adores this stroke!

Friction

Description

Friction movements normally make use of the balls of the thumbs (although fingertips, knuckles or even elbows may be used). The muscle is moved against the bone by small circular movements of the balls of the

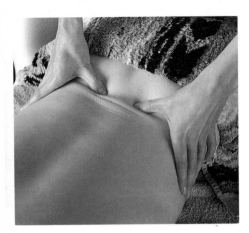

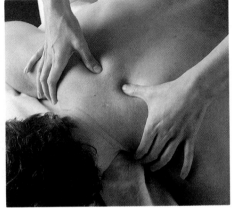

thumbs. Use your body weight to penetrate right down into the deeper tissues – the body is not as delicate and fragile as you might imagine! This stroke is particularly effective when performed on either side of the spine. As a beginner, if your thumbs are not aching by the time you reach the top of the spine you are not performing the stroke correctly!

Benefits

This stroke is particularly useful for breaking down the knots and nodules which build up in the body due to the stresses and strains of daily life. Any accumulated waste products may also be eliminated. Friction helps to break down fatty deposits and is therefore of benefit in cases of obesity. It is also helpful for breaking down *old* scar tissue perhaps from an injury.

Errors to avoid

1 Work deeper and deeper into the tissue *gradually* as pain tolerance levels vary greatly. Do not prod the body indiscriminately.

2 Do not hunch your shoulders with the effort (otherwise you will need a massage straight afterwards!).

Kneading (picking-up/wringing)

Description

This stroke is also referred to as petrissage – the derivation *pétrir* meaning to knead. Kneading can be sub-divided into picking-up, rolling and wringing. If you are good at kneading dough then you will be an expert!

It is an extremely powerful and vigorous movement which enables you to work deeply on the muscles. It may be applied to every area of the

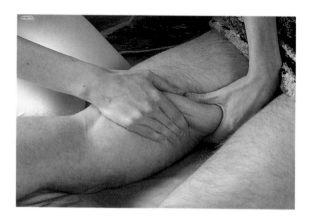

body except for the face, and is very effective on the fleshy areas such as the hips and thighs. In picking-up, the hands are placed flat on the part being treated and the muscle (not the skin) is grasped firmly with both hands and pulled as far away as possible from the bone. Once the muscle has been picked up it may be rolled in both directions – the thumbs may roll the muscle towards the fingers or the fingers may roll the muscle towards the thumbs. Wringing is a variation on picking-up. It is picking-up with a twist! The muscle is picked up and then pulled towards you and 'wrung' out. Imagine that you are wringing out a towel.

Benefits

Kneading has numerous beneficial effects. An increased blood supply is brought to the muscles being worked on, so if you notice a redness and a rise in temperature don't panic as this is caused by the blood flowing into the area and indicates that the action is being performed effectively. This blood brings fresh nutrients to the muscles and any toxins that have accumulated are removed from the deeper tissues. It is valuable in helping to break down and remove fatty deposits around the thighs. It also helps to prevent stiffness from occurring in muscles after exercise.

Errors to avoid

1 Make sure that the whole of the hand is used rather than just the fingers and the thumbs.

2 Pick up the muscle and *not* the skin otherwise there is a danger of pinching.

Percussion movements

Description

Two of the main percussion strokes are 'cupping' and 'hacking' and they may be performed on many areas of the body although they are especially effective when used on fleshy areas such as the thighs.

Cupping is performed with the palms facing downwards and forming a hollow curve. As the cupped hands are brought down onto the body a vacuum is created which is quickly released as the hands are brought up. The sound should be hollow like a horse trotting.

Hacking is probably the most well-known massage stroke since it is the movement almost always shown in the films! It is achieved with the edge of the hands, which are held with the palms facing each other, the thumbs uppermost. They are flicked rhythmically up and down in rapid succession. Use these movements at the end of a massage to wake the person up! Obviously if you are trying to relax someone totally they may be omitted altogether. If you are nervous about using these movements they may first be practised on a cushion. Hacking should be light and bouncy rather than heavy and chopping.

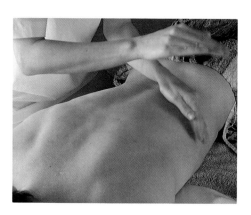 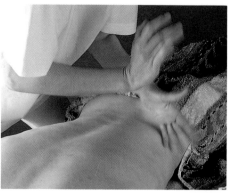

Benefits

Cupping and hacking have the opposite effect to effleurage. Percussion strokes are stimulating, and as the blood is drawn to the surface the circulation is improved. Cupping is very beneficial when performed over the upper and middle back area as it loosens mucus in the lungs, aiding expectoration – in fact it is used in orthodox medicine by physiotherapists for this purpose (postural drainage).

These movements are also valuable in improving muscle tone on flabby and fleshy muscle areas since they stimulate the muscle to contract.

Errors to avoid

1 Make sure that when cupping, the hands are really cupped, otherwise a smacking sensation will be felt, which is painful!

2 When hacking, do not tense up the fingers of the hands or the wrists, otherwise the movements will feel like a karate chop!

3 Keep the hands relaxed and loose and ensure that the movements are coming from the wrist. Keep the elbows tucked closely in, for if you use your elbows and shoulders you will be quickly exhausted.

4 These strokes must *not* be performed over bony areas, bruises or broken veins – they will hurt!

5 Try *not* to concentrate on the strokes otherwise you may lose the rhythm.

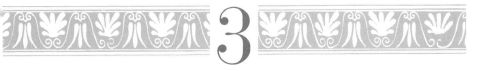

3

STEP-BY-STEP GUIDE TO GIVING A MASSAGE

Having set the scene and prepared the room as detailed in Chapter 1 you are now ready to begin the massage sequence. At the beginning of each section you will find a clearly labelled diagram of the bones and muscles of the area on which you are working followed by any contraindications which must be observed. If your intention is to practise massage professionally, I urge you to train at an establishment where a thorough training in anatomy and physiology is given. (See Useful Addresses.)

Back of the body

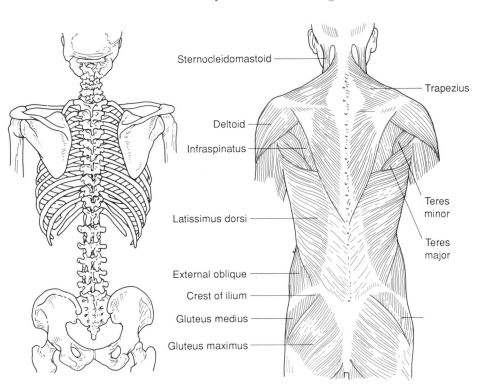

Sternocleidomastoid

Trapezius

Deltoid

Infraspinatus

Teres minor

Teres major

Latissimus dorsi

External oblique

Crest of ilium

Gluteus medius

Gluteus maximus

Don't!

- Work on infectious skin conditions.
- Work directly over recent scar tissue.
- Work on inflamed or swollen areas.
- Use heavy pressure on the lower back of a pregnant woman.

Back and shoulders

We will commence on the back and shoulders since these are areas where most people have problems. Stress (physical or emotional), bad posture, carrying children around, too much gardening or sport and so on are all contributory factors to a tense and knotted back. Massage will afford tremendous relief.

The receiver should lie on the stomach with one pillow placed under the feet, one under the head and shoulders and one under the abdomen, if desired. The arms may be placed at the sides or may hang over the edge of the massage couch. The head may be turned to one side or, if this causes pain, the forehead placed on the hands. Ensure that the receiver is totally covered with towels. Place both hands on the back and take a few deep breaths allowing your own tension to release before you begin. Tune in.

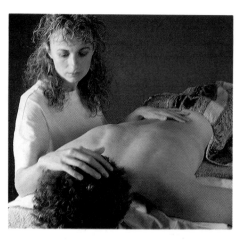

the shoulders. To achieve firm pressure lean into the movement so that your whole body is involved rather than just the hands.

As your hands reach the top of the back spread them outwards across the shoulders.

To complete the movement, allow your hands to glide without

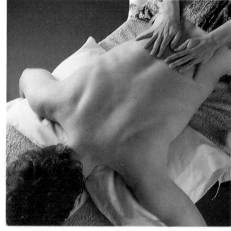

Step 1
Position yourself to one side of the receiver, draw back the towel and begin to oil using the stroking (effleurage) movements.
Commence with both hands on the lower back, one hand either side of the spine, fingers pointing towards the head, and stroke up towards

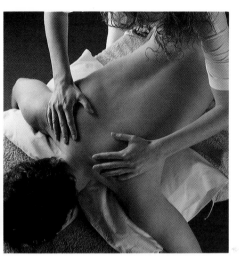

on either side of (but not directly onto) the spine. Start at the base of the spine where you should be able to see two dimples and proceed up as far as the neck. Work with small, slow, firm, deep circular movements using your body weight for greater penetration. Ensure that you maintain the same distance between the thumbs all the time as you travel up the back.

On reaching the neck let your hands return to the starting point with a featherlight touch.

You will be amazed by the number of knots and nodules that you will find even in a seemingly perfectly 'normal' back. This movement will definitely make the beginner's thumbs ache but *do* persevere as it is extremely effective.

any pressure back to your starting point. Breathe out as you stroke up the spine, breathe in as your hands draw back. Repeat this stroking several times to relax the receiver, to establish your own rhythm and to accustom the receiver to your hands. Close your eyes to heighten sensitivity and increase awareness. Try to be aware of any areas of tension, changes in temperature and so forth.

Step 2
Using the balls of the thumbs perform the friction movements

Step 3
Repeat your stroking movements to soothe the receiver and to take away waste products.

Step 4

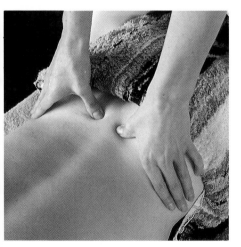

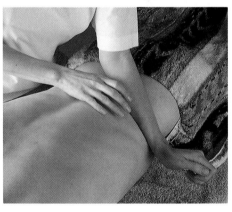

Work up one side of the receiver's back with pushing, ironing-type movements using alternate hands, one hand following closely behind the other. Start from the buttocks area up and over the shoulder and back down again. Take care not to work directly on the spine itself.

Without losing contact, repeat on the other side.

Step 5 – lower back

Place both hands in the middle of the lower back. Stroke firmly out and down over the buttocks. Glide the hands smoothly back.

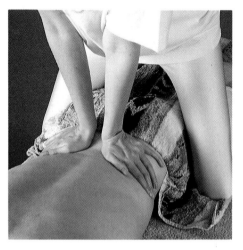

Step 6

Locate the dimples again and with the thumbs use deep circular friction movements around the sacrum (large triangular bone) and across the top of the pelvis.

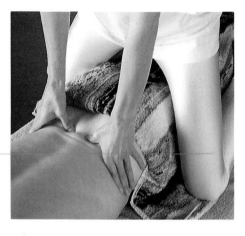

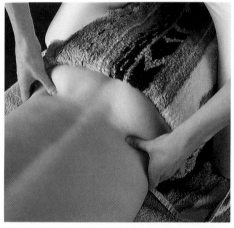

Step 7

Knead the buttock muscles and the waist area using the picking up and wringing movements. Pick up and squeeze the flesh with one hand and bring it towards you. Repeat with the other hand, ensuring that you do not pinch. This is just like making dough!

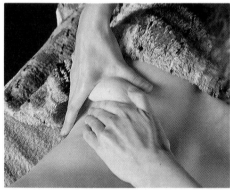

Step 8 – shoulders

Stroke up towards the shoulder area. Bring the towel up with you so that the lower back is covered. Remember that you only expose the area which you are treating.

Step 9

Place one hand flat on top of the other hand and using the whole of

he hand make large circular
movements on and around the
houlder blade. This will warm and
oosen the area.

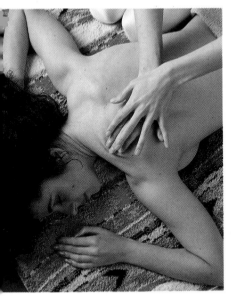

Step 10
The receiver should bend and
place the arm behind the back, if
comfortable. This will make it
easier for you to see the shoulder
blade. Apply deep, circular friction
movements all around the outside
of the shoulder blade. You will
encounter many knots and nodules
n this area.

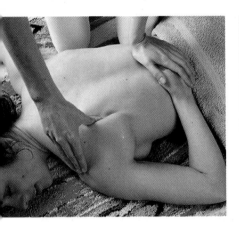

**Repeat steps 9 and 10 on the other
shoulder.**

Step 11

You should return the arms back
to the side. Work across the
shoulders employing the wringing
movements, rhythmically
squeezing and bringing the flesh
towards you with alternate hands.

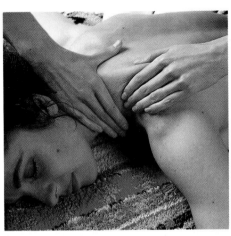

Step 12 – neck
Ask the receiver to place the
forehead onto the hands so as to
straighten the back of the neck. A
small towel may be rolled up and
placed under the forehead for
extra comfort. Pick up and squeeze

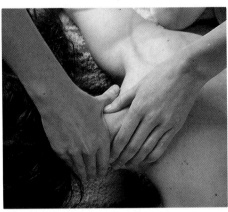

the neck. Grasp and squeeze the muscles either side of the neck **slowly** and **gently** using alternate hands.

Step 13
Position yourself at the receiver's head and firmly stroke the whole back, pushing down and then over the buttock area.

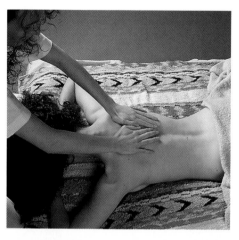

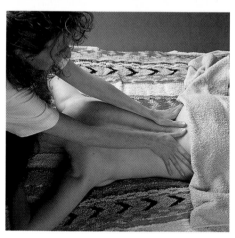

Step 14
Return to the side and cup and hack the back muscles, paying particular attention to the fleshy areas around the buttocks and waist, as these movements help to break down fatty deposits.

Remember that these movements should not be performed directly over bony areas. Cupping and hacking are very effective on the thoracic area for loosening and eliminating mucus from the lungs and bronchial tubes.

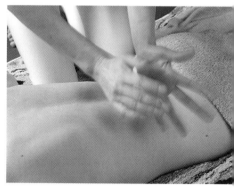

Step 15
With both hands stroke slowly and very gently up either side of the spine using just the fingertips. As you repeat this movement, gradually use lighter and lighter pressure.

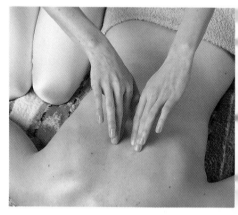

Step 16
Completely cover the lower back with towels and finish by placing both hands intuitively onto the back.

Back of the legs

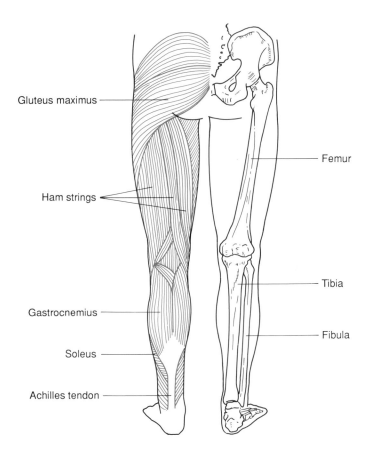

Gluteus maximus

Femur

Ham strings

Tibia

Gastrocnemius

Fibula

Soleus

Achilles tendon

Don't!

* Use heavy pressure over varicose veins as this will aggravate them.
  Very gentle stroking is sufficient.

Leg massage is of great benefit particularly after standing all day at work or after unwisely wearing high heels! It will improve the circulation and thus prevent the arrival of varicose veins. It is also excellent for the lymphatic system. You will observe that sometimes there is swelling at the back of the knee (where there are lymph nodes) and also at the ankles. We always massage *up* the legs towards the lymph glands in the groin area to reduce this fluid. Treatment of the back of the legs helps to alleviate problems in the lower back. Tightness in the upper thigh muscles is usually linked with low back pain. Leg massage is also useful both as a prelude to exercise and afterwards to prevent stiffness.

To tune into the legs place one hand on each calf and take a few deep breaths.

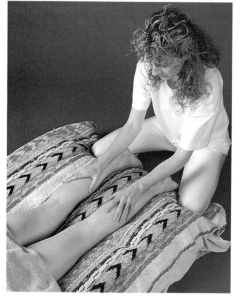

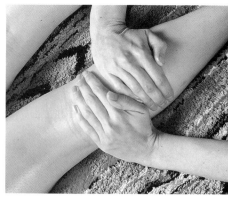

Step 2

Place cupped hands over the back of the ankle, one hand above the other. Stroke up the calf muscles to the back of the knee.

Step 1

Kneel at the feet and stroke from the ankle to the top of the thigh. Hold the hands in a V-shape, one hand in front of the other, moulding your hands to the leg and with most of the pressure on the palms of the hands.

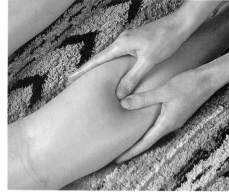

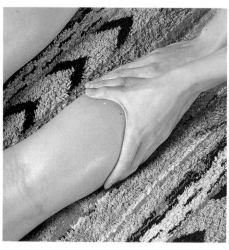

Separate the hands and glide them gently down the sides of the leg to the ankle with no pressure.

Step 3

Using both thumbs apply firm pressure to the calf working from the ankle to just below the back of the knee, and glide back down to the ankle.

Step 4

Position yourself at the side of the calf. Place both hands flat down on the calf muscle ensuring that you use the whole hand to avoid pinching. Pick up and firmly squeeze the muscle (not the skin) with both hands and release.

Step 6

Wring the calf muscles. Pick up and squeeze the muscle with one hand and bring it towards you and repeat with the other hand. These kneading movements on the calf will relax any contraction in the muscles, remove any waste deposits, increase the blood supply and lymph flow and assist in the breaking down of fatty deposits.

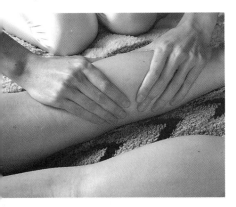

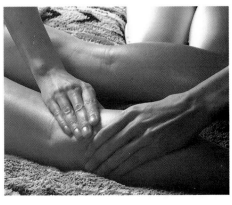

Step 5

Pick up and squeeze the muscle and now, using the thumbs, roll the muscle towards the fingers. Then roll the muscle with the fingers in the other direction towards the thumbs.

Step 7

Stroke the entire leg again towards the heart to move any waste deposits which have been released into the lymph glands in the groin.

Step 8

Firmly stroke the thigh only – firm pressure on the way up, featherlight touch on the return.

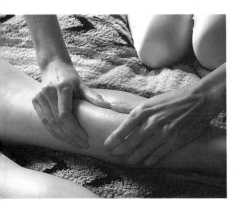

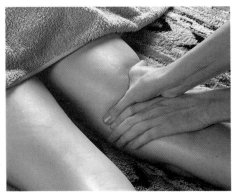

Step 9
Wring the inner thigh muscle by picking up, squeezing and bringing the muscle towards you using alternate hands. Wring the middle thigh muscle.

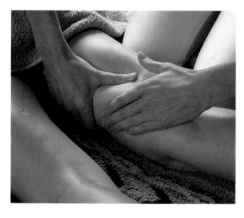

Step 10

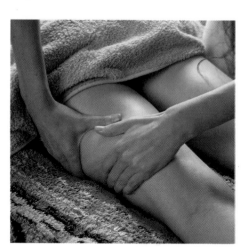

Wring the outer thigh area. This area may be wrung out very firmly since there is usually a generous expanse of flesh where fatty deposits collect and accumulate.

Step 11
Cup and hack over the entire leg taking care to avoid the back of the knee which may be tender. Obviously *do not* perform these actions over varicose veins.

Step 12 ·
Stroke up the whole leg and glide back. Gradually lessen the pressure with each stroke. Let your hands come to rest on the foot. Lift them slowly and gently away.

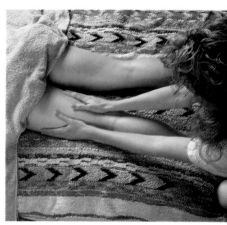

Repeat on the other leg.

Front of the body

Ask the receiver to turn over. Place one pillow under the head and one under the knees. Check for relaxation and comfort.

eet

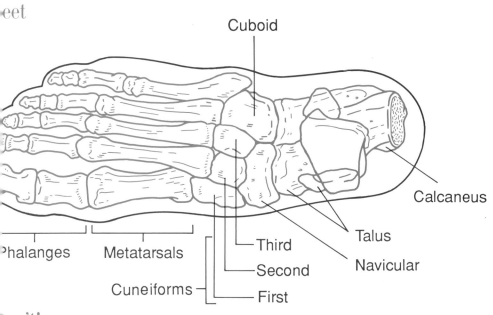

Cuboid

Calcaneus

Phalanges   Metatarsals

Cuneiforms

Third

Second

First

Talus

Navicular

Don't!

Massage directly onto contagious skin conditions – e.g. athlete's foot, verrucas.

Massage firmly onto corns or blisters if this causes pain.

Use too much oil or some of the movements will be impossible to perform.

To tune in, place one hand on the sole of the foot, one hand on top of the foot and take a few deep breaths.

Step 1

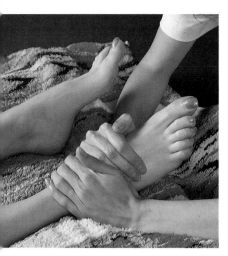

Stroke the entire foot firmly using both hands from the ends of the toes to the top of the foot. Slide around the ankle bones and glide back.

Step 2

Supporting the foot with one hand, massage the entire sole of the foot with the thumb using very firm circular friction movements. Start underneath the ball of the foot and work outwards. Continue to work the rest of the sole in horizontal strips until the whole area has been covered.

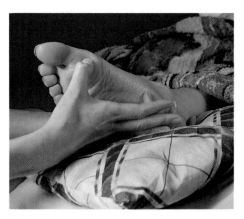

Step 3 – toes

- Slowly stretch each toe individually.

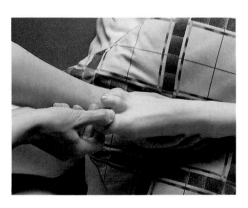

- Massage the joints of the toes, both top and bottom, using the small circular friction movements to loosen them.

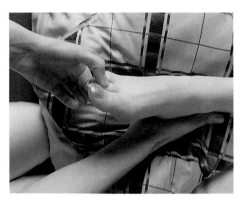

- Hold all the toes in one hand and flex and extend them together.

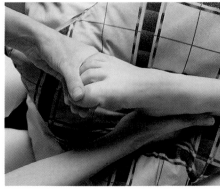

- Rotate each toe individually clockwise and anti-clockwise.

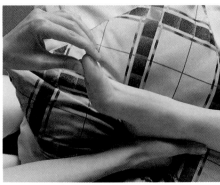

Step 4
Stroke upwards towards the ankle.

Step 5 – ankle

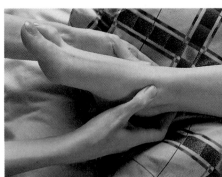

- Massage all around the ankle joint with both thumbs using small, deep, circular friction movements.

- Supporting the foot with one hand, slowly but firmly flex the foot and extend it. This will stretch the Achilles' tendon. It should be performed carefully and cautiously where there is a chronic problem with the tendon.

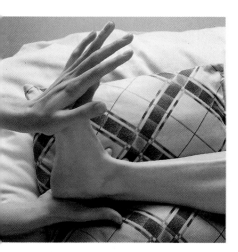

- Move the foot from side to side.

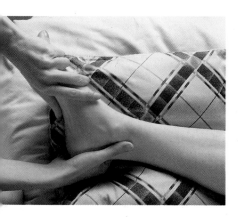

- Rotate the ankle clockwise and anti-clockwise.

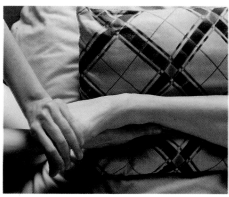

Step 6

Place the palms of your hands, one on each side of the foot, and move them alternately and rapidly from side to side so that the foot vibrates.

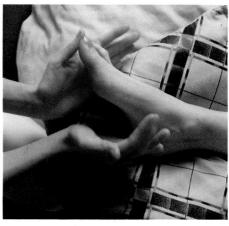

Step 7

Stroke the foot slowly and firmly up towards the ankle.

Front of the legs

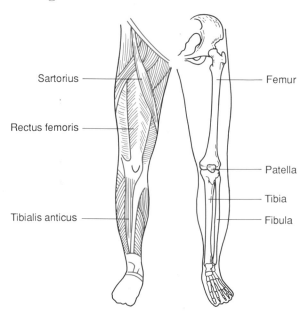

Sartorius

Rectus femoris

Tibialis anticus

Femur

Patella

Tibia

Fibula

Don't!

- Massage on swollen and inflamed joints.

- Massage directly onto varicose veins.

- Perform heavy movements on the lower leg, as this is bony and therefore a delicate area.

Step 1

Position yourself at the receiver's feet. Stroke up the leg from the ankle to the top of the thigh using only light pressure over the knee, moulding your hands to the contours of the leg. Cup your hands over the front of the ankle, one hand above the other and as you reach the top of the thigh, separate the hands and glide them gently down the sides.

Step 2

Stroke the lower half of the leg with cupped hands, from ankle to knee. Use only very gentle pressure on this bony, tender area.

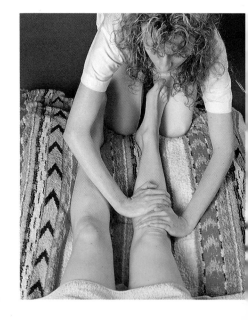

Step 3

Work all around the knee cap with the thumbs using small, circular friction movements.

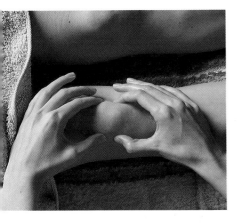

Step 4

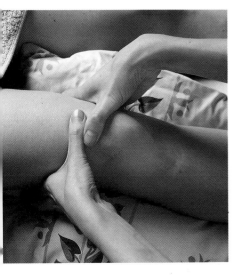

To complete the knee commence with both thumbs under the knee cap and glide both thumbs around the knee until they meet each other at the top. Glide them to meet at the bottom.

Step 5

Firmly stroke the front of the thigh.

Step 6

Pick up, roll and wring the inner thigh muscles. Wring the middle muscles and outer thigh.

Step 7

Cup and hack over the muscles of the thigh *only*. Do *not* cup and hack over the lower leg as this will cause pain on such a bony area.

Step 8

Stroke up the whole of the leg several times, gradually decreasing the pressure until your hands come to rest gently back on the foot.

Repeat the foot and leg movements on the other side.

Abdomen

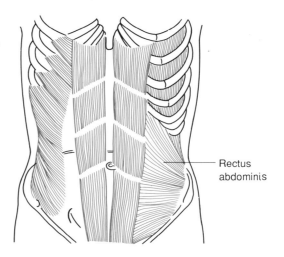

Rectus
abdominis

Don't!

- Massage the abdomen *firmly* during pregnancy.

- Massage over *recent* scar tissue.

- Massage the abdomen immediately after a heavy meal.

- Massage when there is an inflammatory condition e.g. gastritis.

Having the abdomen massaged is a wonderful and very beneficial experience. It is not only relaxing and soothing but it is marvellous for constipation and fluid retention. Some people may be sensitive about having the abdomen touched but they are always pleasantly surprised.

To tune in place your hands flat down, one on top of the other, on the navel and take a few deep breaths.

Step 1
Position yourself on the right-hand side of the receiver because then you are able to follow the colon in the appropriate direction. Begin with a small circular motion, one hand on top of the other, moving in a *clockwise* direction gradually increasing in size. Employ very gentle pressure, gradually increasing the depth and intensity with each movement.

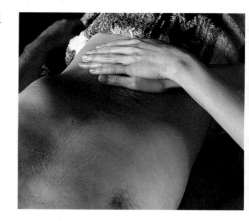

Step 2

Perform circular stroking, moving in a *clockwise* direction around the abdomen using both hands at the same time, one hand following behind the other.

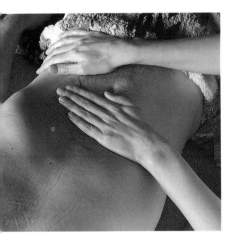

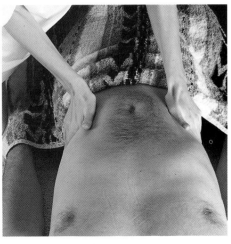

Step 3

Stroke and pull up around the side of the waist using both hands.

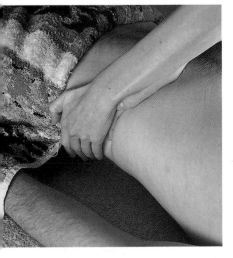

Repeat on the other side of the waist. Repeat pulling up on both sides at the same time, allowing your fingers to meet under the receiver's waist.

Step 4

Wring the waist and hip area with alternate hands, squeezing and pulling the flesh towards you.

Step 5

To work on the colon begin at the bottom right-hand side of the abdomen. With the three middle fingers of one hand perform small circular movements working up the ascending colon (top right-hand side) across the transverse colon and down the descending colon (bottom left-hand side).

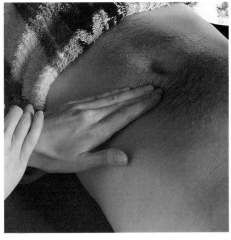

Step 6

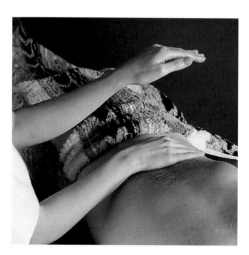

Cup and hack the waist and hip area on both sides of the body to increase muscle tone and to break down fatty deposits.

Step 7

Repeat the clockwise circular stroking, working smoothly with one hand following the other. Gradually decrease the pressure until you are scarcely touching the skin.

Step 8

Finish with both hands resting on the navel.

Arm and hand

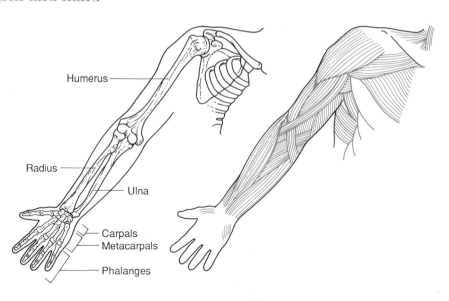

Humerus

Radius

Ulna

Carpals
Metacarpals

Phalanges

Don't!

● Massage over inflamed joints.

To tune in place both hands on the arm and breathe deeply in and out.

Step 1

Position yourself at the side of the receiver and place the arm slightly away from the body to allow easier access. Support under the forearm with one hand as you firmly stroke up the arm from the wrist to the

houlder. On reaching the top
lide lightly back down the sides.

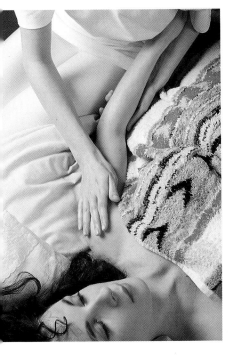

Step 2
Work with slow, circular friction
movements around the front and
op of the shoulder to loosen and
mobilise it.

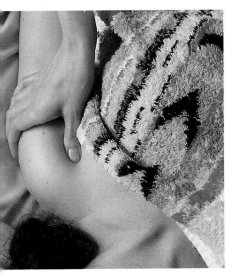

Step 3
Place one hand under the elbow
and the other hand around the
shoulder. Lift the arm and **gently**
rotate it clockwise and anti-
clockwise.

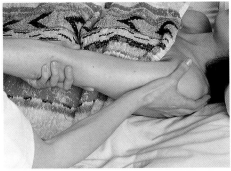

Step 4
Working with both hands wring
the muscles of the upper arm.

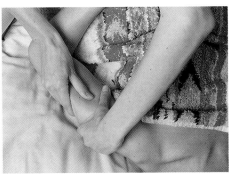

Step 5 – elbow

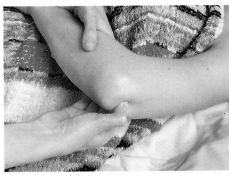

Support the arm with one hand and use the circular friction movements all around the elbow to loosen and mobilise.

Step 6

Place one hand on top of the upper arm, and with the other hand take the elbow gently and slowly into flexion and extension.

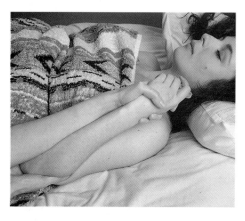

Step 7

Stroke the forearm firmly from the wrist to the elbow leaving the upper arm down and lifting up the

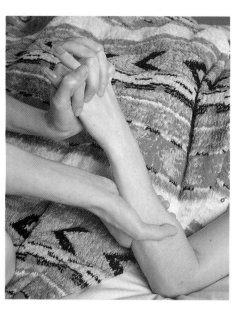

forearm. Hold the wrist with one hand whilst stroking with the other.

Step 8 – wrist

Use the thumbs to friction with small circular movements around the wrist.

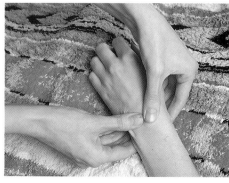

Step 9

Interlock your fingers with the receiver and bend the wrist backwards and forwards, side to

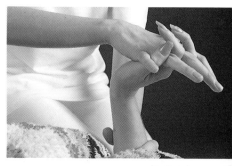

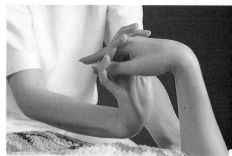

side and rotate it clockwise and anti-clockwise.

Step 10

Work into the palm of the hand with circular movements with a clenched fist to loosen muscles, tendons and joints.

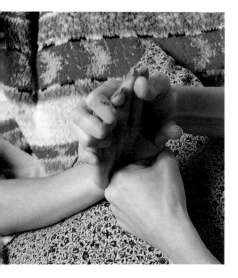

Step 11

Stroke across the back of the hand using both thumbs. Rest your fingertips in the palm of the receiver's hand.

Step 12 – fingers

- Gently and slowly squeeze and stretch each finger individually.

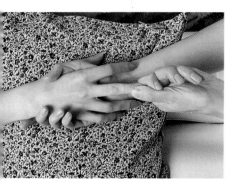

- Friction the fingers with thumb and index finger to loosen.

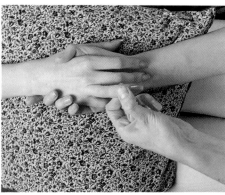

- Flex and extend each finger.

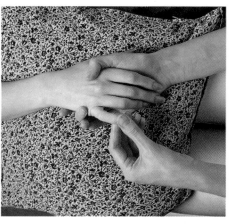

- Circle the fingers individually both ways.

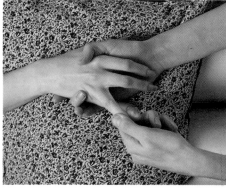

Step 13
Stroke firmly up the arm from
fingers to shoulder. Glide back.
Lighten the movement until there
is virtually no pressure at all.

Step 14
On the final stroke clasp the
receiver's hand between both of
your hands and squeeze gently.

Repeat on the other arm and hand.

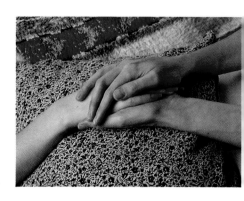

Upper chest and neck

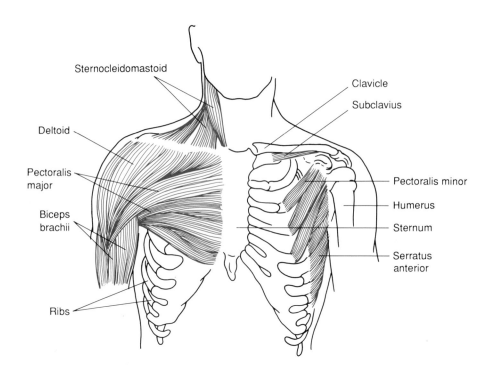

Don't!

- Apply too much pressure to these delicate and sensitive areas.

Position yourself at the receiver's head. To tune in rest your hands on top
of the shoulders and take a few deep breaths.

Step 1
Commence at the centre of the chest. Bend and relax the fingers and with the back of both hands stroke gently outwards towards the armpits. As you reach the shoulders turn the hands over and use the palms to stroke and direct the lymph into the glands under the arms.

Make *gentle* circular movements with either the fingers or knuckles starting at the centre of the chest, working towards and around the front of the shoulders.

Step 3
Turn the head to the side. Place one hand on the temple and stroke *one* hand down the side of the neck and over the shoulder. Glide the hand lightly back.

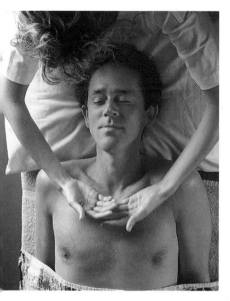

Step 2

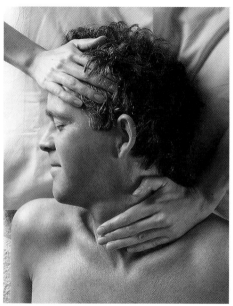

Repeat on the other side of the neck. These movements are excellent for removing tension away from the neck and thus preventing or relieving headaches and migraines.

Step 4
To stretch the neck, cup both hands under the head with the fingers at the base of the skull. Pull gently and slowly towards you as you lean backwards, thus using your own body weight to traction the neck. Breathe out as you

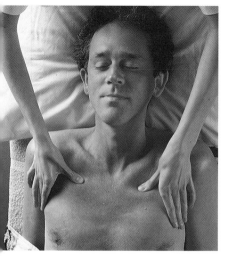

stretch the neck and in as you
gradually release the stretch.

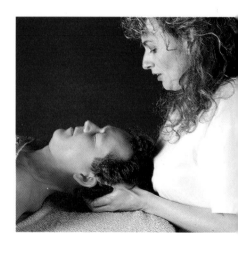

Face and scalp

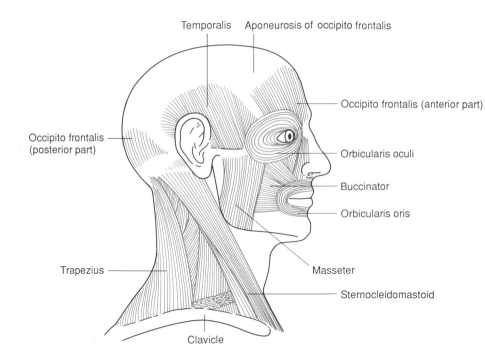

Temporalis   Aponeurosis of occipito frontalis

Occipito frontalis (anterior part)

Occipito frontalis
(posterior part)

Orbicularis oculi

Buccinator

Orbicularis oris

Trapezius

Masseter

Sternocleidomastoid

Clavicle

Don't!

- Apply too much oil to the face.
- Massage over contact lenses.

To tune in, place both hands almost without touching onto the forehead
and breathe deeply.

Step 1
Stroke out across the forehead using fingertips and glide back with feather light touch.

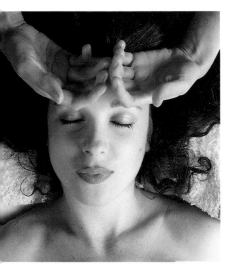

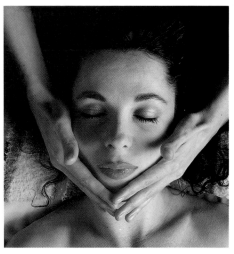

Step 4
Stroke the forehead firmly with both thumbs, working from the centre of the forehead outwards and commencing just above the eyebrows. Work up the forehead in horizontal strips covering the whole forehead up as far as the hairline.

Step 2
Stroke down the sides of the nose and out across the cheeks.

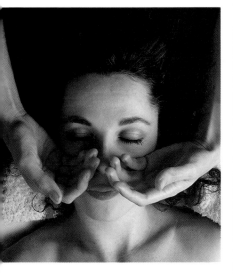

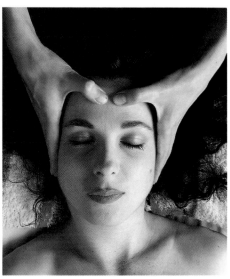

Step 3
Stroke outwards across the chin and continue stroking down the neck, towards the shoulders.

These movements are effective for relieving headaches and tension.

Step 5

Using both thumbs stroke down the sides of the nose. This is excellent for sinusitis and blocked up nasal passages!

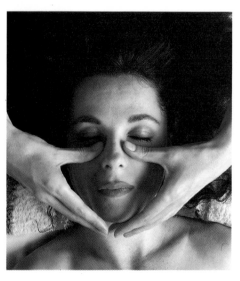

Step 7

Commence just under the mouth and with the thumbs stroke outwards covering the entire chin and jaw area.

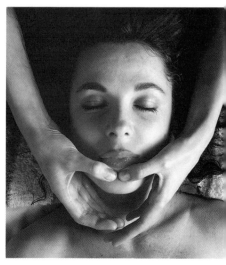

Step 6

Commence under the eyes and with the thumbs stroke across the cheeks to the sides of the face. Cover the whole of the cheek area and as you reach the ears stretch and release them gently.

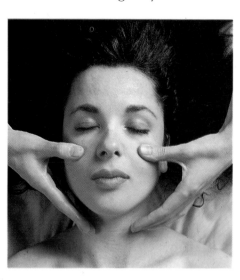

Step 8 – scalp

Glide your hands gently up towards the scalp. Using the fingertips press firmly into the scalp making small, circular

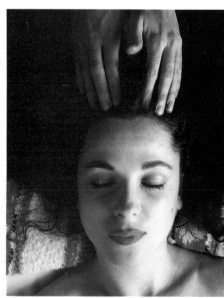

friction movements. You should be able to feel the skin moving under your fingers. Cover the entire scalp.

Step 9
Stroke the hair gently to release the last remaining tension and gradually let your hands come to rest on the temples.

Massage sequence memory jogger

Back of the body

The back
Tune in.

1 Stroke up the whole back.
2 Friction on either side of the spine.
3 Stroke whole back.
4 Pushing/ironing down both sides of the back.
5 Stroke lower back.
6 Friction around sacrum and across top of pelvis.
7 Knead buttocks and waist area.
8 Stroke shoulder area.
9 Friction around each shoulder blade.
10 Wring across the top of the shoulders.
11 Pick up the neck.
12 Stroke down the whole back.
13 Cupping and hacking.
14 Stroke up the whole back.

Backs of the legs
Tune in.

1 Stroke up the whole leg (V-Shape).
2 Stroke the lower leg (cupped hands).
3 Thumbs up back of lower leg.
4 Pick up and squeeze lower leg.
5 Pick up and roll lower leg (both ways).
6 Wring lower leg.
7 Stroke up the whole leg.
8 Firmly stroke the thigh.
9 Wring inner and middle thigh.
10 Wring outer thigh.
11 Cup and hack whole leg.
12 Stroke the whole leg.

Repeat on other leg.

Front of the body

Feet and the front of the legs
Tune in.

1 Stroke up the whole foot.
2 Friction the sole of the foot.
3 Toes – stretch, friction, flex and extend, rotate in both directions.
4 Stroke up to the ankle.

5 Ankle – friction, flex and extend, side to side, rotate in both directions.

6 Vibrate the foot rapidly from side to side.

7 Stroke up the whole foot.

8 Stroke up the whole leg.

9 Stroke up lower leg.

10 Friction around knee.

11 Circular gliding around knee.

12 Stroke up thigh.

13 Wring inner, middle and outer thigh.

14 Cup and hack thigh *only*.

15 Stroke up the whole leg.

Repeat on other foot and leg.

Abdomen
Tune in.

1 Two handed circling.

2 Circular stroking in clockwise direction.

3 Pulling up the sides of the waist.

4 Wring waist and hip area.

5 Colon massage.

6 Cup and hack waist and hip area.

7 Circular stroking.

Arm and hand
Tune in.

1 Stroke up the whole arm.

2 Friction shoulder.

3 Rotate arm in both directions.

4 Wring upper arm muscles.

5 Friction elbow.

6 Flex and extend elbow.

7 Stroke up forearm.

8 Friction wrist.

9 Bend wrist backwards and forwards, side to side, rotate clockwise and anti-clockwise.

10 Friction palm.

11 Stroke back of hand.

12 Fingers – squeeze and stretch, friction, flex and extend, circle.

13 Stroke up the whole arm.

14 Squeeze hand gently.

Upper chest and neck
Tune in.

1 Stroke across chest towards the armpits.

2 Circular finger knuckle movements towards the armpits.

3 Stroke down the neck one side. Repeat on the other side.

4 Stretch the neck.

Face and scalp
Tune in.

1 Stroke forehead, cheeks and chin.

2 Stroke across forehead with thumbs.

3 Stroke down both sides of nose.

4 Stroke across cheeks and stretch ears.

5 Stroke outwards across chin.

6 Circular friction to scalp.

7 Stroke hair.

8 Rest hands on temples.

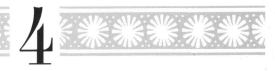

4

AROMATHERAPY AND MASSAGE

A brief history

The history of the use of aromatic oils employed in a healing context is documented as long ago as four and a half thousand years BC. In ancient Egypt aromatics were a part of daily life, commonly used for embalming the dead, in religious ceremonies, as perfume and as medicines.

There are many historical references to the therapeutic use of essential oils. In the Middle Ages, for example, it is related that during cholera and other epidemics those who worked with essential oils enjoyed immunity from disease. Lavender was widely used to protect against infection.

The rediscovery of essential oils is accredited to the French biochemist Professor R.M. Gattefosse. It is claimed that after burning his hand in an experiment he plunged it into the nearest liquid which happened to be lavender. To his astonishment the burns healed much faster than anticipated, without scarring. During World War One he experimented on soldiers and discovered many oils which greatly accelerated the healing process. His work was continued by the renowned Dr Jean Valnet, one of the leading authorities on aromatherapy. Nowadays the use of essential oils is widespread in both health and beauty care.

Essential oils – what they are and how they work

Essential oils are considered to be the 'hormones', 'life force' or 'soul' of plants. They are extracted from various sources including leaves (**eucalyptus**), flowers (**rose**), grasses (**lemongrass**), fruit (**bergamot**), roots (**ginger**), seeds (**fennel**), wood (**sandalwood**) and so on. Their healing powers may be employed to rejuvenate and regenerate the human body, to relieve the stress of modern living and to enhance well-being. Some oils calm and soothe, relieving stress or nervous-related disorders, whereas others stimulate, to uplift body, mind and spirit. Some oils aid circulation, others rejuvenate the skin and others are used to affect bodily functions such as digestion and menstruation. There are many more benefits. When blended with a carrier oil and applied by massage they reach the blood and lymph where they may be transported to wherever they are required. Used properly they are extremely safe, leaving behind no toxic residues and creating no harmful side effects. Essential oils are an excellent way of enhancing your massage.

Blending and storing

Pure essential oils are highly concentrated and must never be used undiluted for they may be harmful. As a carrier choose any good quality vegetable oil (not mineral oil) and to blend use just **3** to **4** drops of pure essential oil to 2 teaspoons (10 ml) of base oil. Just a few teaspoons should be sufficient for a massage. If you wish to mix a larger quantity of oil then bear in mind that a blended oil only lasts about three months. It is very unlikely that a particular massage blend will suit more than one individual.

Pure essential oils and blended oils must be stored in amber or dark coloured bottles since they are sensitive to ultraviolet light. They evaporate very easily – so do not leave the top off the bottle. Extremes of temperature will also damage pure essential oils. They should be stored in a cool, dark place.

The Top 10 essential oils

It is virtually impossible to choose from the vast range of essential oils. However, I have chosen 10 of the most common and versatile and listed their main properties. These 10 oils will fulfil most of your requirements. It is vital to use only high quality *pure* essential oils. If you find these difficult to obtain then please refer to the *Useful Addresses* section at the back of the book.

For further information on a whole host of other oils and different methods of application you may like to read my other book in this series on *Aromatherapy*.

Chamomile

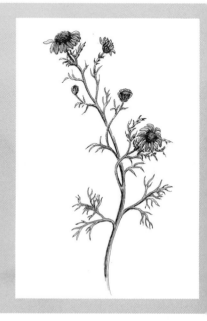

Key words
- Calming, soothing, anti-inflammatory.

Indications
- Particularly suitable for children and sensitive individuals due to its low toxicity.

- All digestive problems, especially where there is inflammation, e.g. colitis (any condition ending in 'itis'!).

- Female disorders, especially where there is nervous tension, e.g. menopause and PMT.

- Aches and pain, whether in muscles, joints or organs, e.g. rheumatism, arthritis, backache, cramp, earache, headache, toothache.

- Sensitive and allergic skin conditions.

- Nervous disorders – depression, insomnia, irritability, impatience, restlessness.

Contraindications
None.

Cypress

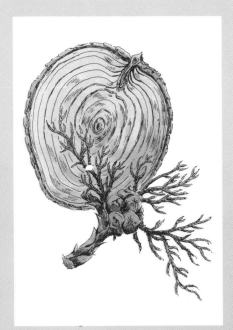

Key words
Reduces fluid, astringent.

Indications
- Fluid retention (of ankles, wrists, etc.).

- Menopause and PMT.

- Oily skin.

- Varicose veins (only very gentle stroking).

- Spasmodic coughs.

Contraindications
None.

Eucalyptus

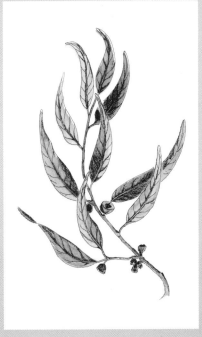

Key words
Relieves coughs and eliminates catarrh. Stimulant. Pain relieving.

Indications
- Excellent as an inhalant and chest rub for all respiratory disorders.
- Throat infections, sinusitis.
- Prevents the spread of contagious diseases.
- Arthritis, muscular and rheumatic pain.

Contraindications
Take care with sensitive skin.

Geranium

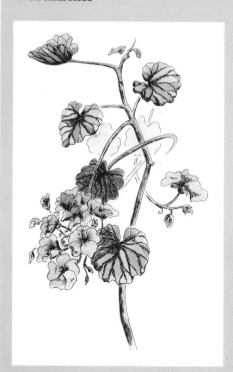

Key words
Balancing – of emotions, hormones, skin, etc.

Indications
- Menopause and PMT.
- Throat infection.
- All anxiety states – sedative yet uplifting.
- All skin types, especially combination skin. It will balance the skin.

Contraindications
None.

Lavender

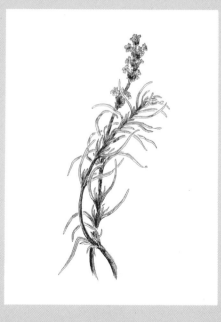

Key words
Most versatile and useful of all essential oils. All conditions.

Indications
- All nervous disorders – anxiety, stress, depression, insomnia, irritability, panics.

- High blood pressure and palpitations.

- All digestive disorders.

- Headache and migraine.

- Muscular aches and pains, arthritis, rheumatism.

- All skin types – even sensitive skin. It rejuvenates and regenerates. Burns, acne, eczema.

- Children and sensitive individuals.

Contraindications
None.

Indications
- All forms of illness. It stimulates the white blood cells to accelerate recovery time.

- All digestive problems, especially where there is acid.

- Sore throat, tonsillitis, laryngitis.

- Colds and coughs.

- Cuts and all skin eruptions (e.g. warts) – apply neat.

- Greasy skin.

Contraindications
Take care with extra sensitive skin.

Lemon

Peppermint

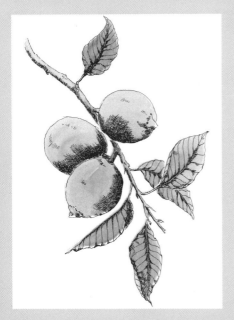

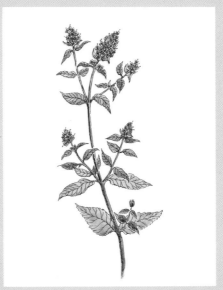

Key words
Antiseptic, alkaline, stimulating.

Key words
Digestive, cooling, pain relieving, stimulant.

Indications
- All digestive problems.
- Headaches and migraine.
- Clears mind – mental fatigue.
- Coughs and colds.
- Sunburn and skin redness.

Contraindications
- Store away from homoeopathic medicines.
- Take care with sensitive skin.

Rosemary

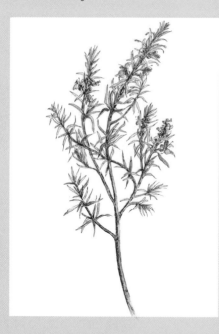

Key words
General debility, muscular problems, stimulant.

Indications
- Loss of function (muscles, memory, hair, etc.).

- Arthritic, rheumatic pains.
- Tired, overworked muscles.
- Coughs and colds.
- Invigorating.

Contraindications
None.

Sandalwood

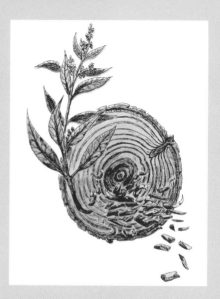

Key words
Relaxing, sedative yet uplifting.

Indications
- Fluid retention.
- Cystitis.
- Sore throat.
- Tension, insomnia, depression.
- All skin care, especially dry.

Contraindications
None.

Tangerine

Key word
Tonic.

Indications
- Children.

- Pregnancy

- Tonic for the stomach.

- Refreshing and revitalising.

- Peripheral circulation.

Contraindications
None.

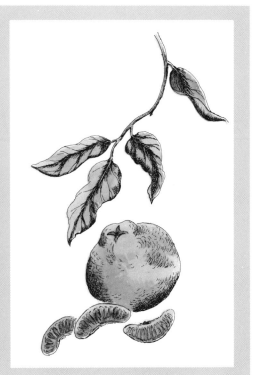

REMEMBER
Do *not* use neat

Use 3 to 4 drops of pure essential oil to 2 teaspoons of base oil.

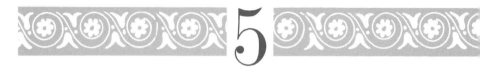

5

THE BACH FLOWER REMEDIES

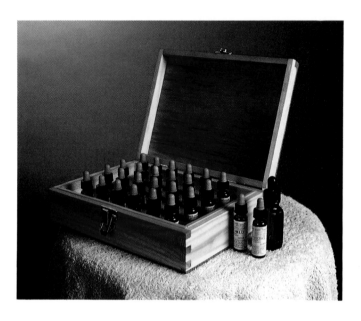

The 38 Bach Flower Remedies are an excellent accompaniment to massage. They provide a method of healing using essences prepared from non-poisonous wild flowers. They are administered internally and can be taken by people of all ages from young babies to the elderly and even by animals and plants. They are non-habit forming, produce no harmful side effects and may be taken alongside all other medicines with no risk of conflict. In my opinion they are of use to every family.

The Remedies were developed in 1930 by a renowned physician Dr Edward Bach who abandoned his highly lucrative Harley Street practice to devote the last six years of his life to a search for a natural method of healing. He had become very disillusioned with the orthodox idea of treating symptoms with medicines that very often resulted in harmful side effects. He felt that he should be treating the person and dealing with the root cause of the problem rather than with its symptoms.

The Bach Flower Remedies aim to establish an equilibrium between mind, body and spirit as it is disharmony which creates disease. Ill health originates in an inharmonious mind. Feelings which are persistently repressed emerge first as mental conflicts. These conflicting moods produce unhappiness which lowers the body's vitality and resistance to lisease and thus the physical illness is allowed to develop. The Remedies reat the person's moods and deal with negative states of mind, such as anger, worry, jealousy or depression, rather than with the symptoms of the physical illness. It is these negative states of mind which are blocking the free flow of the life force and causing the disease. *Once they are treated, balanced health is restored.*

As you massage you will undoubtedly find that many old and unwanted emotions rise to the surface. This often happens with my students at the college, some of whom undergo dramatic transformations on completion of the course. Memories, problems and unresolved issues which are too difficult to deal with lock themselves in the muscles and issues and, as the knots and nodules are released, so are the hidden emotions. Some undergo personality changes and experience thoughts and feelings they have suppressed and have felt unable to deal with before. Fear, guilt, anger, frustration, bitterness, resentment, despair, indecision and many more emotions appear and need to be worked through. The Bach Flower Remedies are a very powerful tool to have at your disposal when dealing with these states of anguish.

The Bach Flower Remedies are available from most health food stores and some chemists.

Preparation of the Remedies

The Bach Flower Remedies may be taken singly or in any combination up to a maximum of six. To prepare a remedy almost fill a 30 ml dropper bottle with pure spring water, add a teaspoon of brandy for preservation purposes and then add 2 drops of what you consider to be the appropriate remedies. The dosage is 4 drops of the diluted Remedy either in a glass of water or straight on the tongue 4 times a day.

The most widely used Remedy which you may have come into contact with is 'Rescue Remedy', a composite of five flower remedies. It contains: **cherry plum** (for desperation), **clematis** (for the out-of-the-body feeling), **impatiens** (for tension), **rock rose** (for panic), **star of Bethlehem** (for shock).

Personally, I always keep a bottle in my handbag for emergency purposes. It can be administered in times of sudden shock, grief, anguish and panic. It is wonderful for relieving apprehension and is beneficial prior to exams, driving tests, going to the dentist and so on. Use it whenever you feel 'tensed up'. It's far better for you than a cigarette!

I do not propose to outline the main uses of all 38 Remedies. I will mention those which I have found to be most useful. If you wish to learn more there are numerous books on the market.

Aspen
- For unknown fear. Such fear descends for no apparent reason usually occurring when the person is alone, filling them with absolute terror.

Centaury
- For the weak-willed, easily taken advantage of person who cannot say 'no'. They are the 'doormats' of society.

Cherry Plum
- For the desperate, perhaps on the verge of a nervous breakdown. They fear that they will lose total control and commit suicide.

Crab Apple
- For feelings of self-disgust. For those who feel unclean and in need of cleansing.

Gorse
- For hopelessness and other despair. Valuable when a person has been suffering for a long time with chronic disease and, having tried many treatments without success, is ready to give up.

Holly
- For jealousy, envy, distrust, suspicion and hatred.

Honeysuckle
- For those longing for the past and unable to live in the present, e.g. a widow or widower clinging to the memory of a lost partner.

Hornbeam
- For that Monday morning feeling.

Impatiens
- For impatience and irritability. Inability to tolerate fools gladly. Anger flaring up quickly and disappearing as quickly as it came.

Larch
- For lack of self-confidence, inferiority complexes.

Mimulus
- For known fear, e.g. fear of cancer, of being alone, flying, lifts, etc.

Mustard
- For bouts of depression and gloom which appear for no reason.

Olive
- For total exhaustion. When you feel sick with exhaustion and so tired you could cry.

Pine
- For self-reproach and guilt.

Red Chestnut
- For excessive worry over others e.g. an over-protective mother worrying about her children.

Schleranthus
- For indecision. Opinions and moods change rapidly.

Vervain
- For the inability to relax physically. Totally keyed up and lives on nerves. Extremely highly strung and usually only sleeps a few hours a night.

Walnut
- For changes. Useful for teething, change of job, change of house, divorce, puberty, pregnancy and menopause.

White Chestnut
- For persistent unwanted thoughts going round and round in the mind. May have problems going to sleep and is woken up early in the morning by thoughts.

Willow
- For resentment. A 'poor-me' attitude. Accepts no personal responsibility and blames others for misfortunes. A victim.

erhaps you may notice a few Remedies which *you* require. The
Remedies will usually act fairly quickly and in the case of babies and
children almost immediately since they have so much energy to work
with. Although I was very sceptical at first, the Remedies never cease to
amaze me. When my son was born for instance, my two-year-old
daughter was overcome with jealousy. After a few doses of **holly** she was
completely cured.

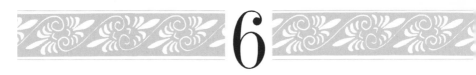

6

MASSAGE FOR COMMON AILMENTS

Massage is essential for the prevention of disease and the promotion of good health and has beneficial effects on *all* the systems of the body. However, when treating common ailments I should like to point out the necessity of always consulting your doctor where problems are persistent or serious. Suggested essential oils in this chapter have been selected from my Top 10. For further, more detailed information on a wide variety of oils and treatment techniques, please consult my other book in this series on *Aromatherapy*.

Circulatory problems

Good circulation is vital to good health, and massage is excellent for improving the functioning of the cardiovascular system (heart and circulation). Useful essential oils to blend with your carrier oil are **lemon** and **rosemary**. Exercise, of course, is also vital.

Varicose veins will also respond positively to massage. More women than men suffer from this complaint which occurs when the valves in the veins are faulty and unable to keep the blood from flowing backwards, resulting in varicosity. The varicose veins often appear in pregnancy, and obesity certainly exacerbates this ailment. The legs will be sore and aching. Many books advise against massaging varicose veins but they can benefit enormously from *gentle* and *careful* stroking. *Never* cup and hack. The legs can be massaged daily with any base oil to which you have added **cypress** and **lemon**. These two essential oils will encourage the blood vessels to contract.

High blood pressure and heart problems

Massage is a well accepted form of therapy for reducing high blood pressure by inducing a deep sense of relaxation. Blood pressure always rises when we are anxious, emotional and stressed-up. Since nutrition is obviously an important factor, a healthy, balanced diet is vital. Particularly avoid salt, sugar, processed foods, fatty foods and too much tea and coffee. Eat plenty of fresh fruit and vegetables. Try to take regular, gentle exercise.

Always use very slow and gentle stroking movements to calm and soothe. Never use brisk, stimulating movements. Essential oils such as **chamomile**, **lavender**, **sandalwood** and **ylang ylang** may be added to your vegetable oil to enhance the relaxation effects.

Digestive problems

Digestive problems often originate from stresses manifesting themselves in the form of indigestion, heartburn, obesity, constipation, diarrhoea and so forth. Since massage relieves tension it is bound to have a beneficial effect on the digestive system. Abdominal massage is even used in some hospitals nowadays for the relief of constipation in preference to drugs. Not only does it carry no risk of side-effects but it is also more effective!

Massage the abdomen whenever necessary, always moving the hands in a clockwise direction. Start gently and gradually increase the pressure. Wait for action! To enhance the effects of the treatment try adding pure essential oils to your base oils. The suggestions I have made include only the 10 essential oils described in this book:

Constipation
- Rosemary.

Diarrhoea
- Chamomile, geranium.

Flatulence
- Chamomile, lavender, lemon, peppermint, rosemary, tangerine.

Heartburn
- Lemon.

Indigestion
- Chamomile, lavender, peppermint, rosemary, tangerine.

Loss of appetite
- Chamomile, peppermint.

Nausea
- Chamomile, lavender, peppermint, rosemary.

Obesity
- Lemon, rosemary.

Stomach pains
- Chamomile, lavender, peppermint, rosemary.

Stomach ulcers
- Chamomile, lemon.

The Bach Flower Remedy, **crab apple**, is often excellent for bowel problems since it is a powerful cleanser.

Genito-urinary problems

Fluid retention

Massage undoubtedly improves the circulation and stimulates lymphatic flow aiding the elimination of toxins and is therefore extremely useful for fluid retention. Oedema (swelling due to fluid retention) is commonly experienced in the elderly, particularly in the ankles and wrists, and massage will reduce the fluid dramatically. Work gently, encouraging the fluid towards the nearest main lymph nodes (back of knee, groin, elbow, armpit, neck). Urge the receiver between treatments to rotate the ankles or wrists daily and, if they are capable, to massage themselves.

Essential oils for fluid retention include: **cypress** (particularly good), **eucalyptus**, **geranium**, **lavender**, **lemon**, **rosemary** and **sandalwood**.

Menstrual problems

Massage of the lower back and the abdomen with **lavender** will help to alleviate menstrual pain. **Peppermint** is renowned for its analgesic properties and just one drop of peppermint oil in a glass of water is as effective as an aspirin. Compresses of **lavender** and **peppermint** on the lower back and abdomen may be useful. Where there is fluid retention a combination of **lavender** and **cypress** can be blended. Both premenstrual and menopausal women may be effectively treated with **chamomile** and **geranium**. **Chamomile** is soothing and **geranium** helps to balance the hormones. As it is sedative, yet at the same time uplifting, it will ease the feelings of irritability and depression experienced by many women. I have many patients who have found that by having a full body massage once a month their PMT has completely gone. Breast tenderness which is often experienced prior to menstruation, may be relieved by massaging this area with a **geranium** blend.

The Bach Flower Remedy, **walnut**, is particularly indicated for the menopause since it is the Remedy for transition and change. **Impatiens** may be employed for the impatience and irritability which is present where there are menstrual problems, especially premenstrual tension. **Olive** will help to combat exhaustion and tiredness.

Muscular/skeletal problems

Arthritis

Osteo-arthritis is a degenerative joint disease caused by wear and tear and is usually considered to be part of the ageing process generally occurring in the over fifties. It mostly affects the weight-bearing joints of the body such as the knees and hips, limiting movement and is definitely worsened by being over-weight. It is vital to keep the joints as mobile as possible and massage is ideal for this purpose.

Rheumatoid arthritis can affect any and every joint in the body but particularly involves the wrists and fingers, resulting eventually in a 'cigar-like' appearance of the fingers. It is a painful, disabling condition occurring most commonly between the ages of 40 and 60 years but may affect people at any age. Even children may be subject to this ailment. The cause is unknown, although it is believed to be an auto-immune disease – the body attacks itself. Sufferers may have remissions at any time.

The common complaint is a burning sensation with swelling. The intensity of the disease is variable with some days being much worse than others and the disease can start in one joint, remain there for a long time and then for no apparent reason spread to other joints. When the joints are very painful and inflamed, massage is contraindicated. However, once the inflammation has subsided, massage can be applied.

Diet is a major factor in the prevention and alleviation of arthritic conditions. The consumption of highly processed and over-cooked food leads to a build-up of toxic waste which is not expelled and damages internal organs and erodes joints. Many find great relief when they eliminate or reduce dairy foods, sugar, red meat, tea and coffee. The emphasis should be on an increase in the consumption of *fresh* fruit and vegetables from which *all* the necessary vitamins and minerals may be derived. A glass of warm water on rising with half a freshly squeezed lemon in it is often found to be helpful.

In cases of arthritis where the receiver is elderly, it will sometimes not be comfortable to give a massage on the floor or couch. A chair may be used instead. Older people often prefer as far as possible to keep their clothes on and so you must be prepared to roll garments up and to work through clothing. On the elderly, use fairly gentle pressure as the skin

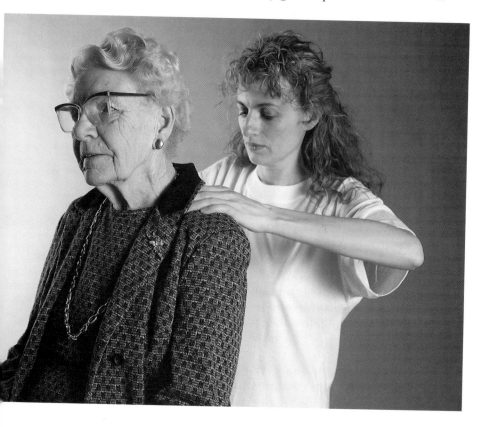

tends to be thinner and sensitivity is greater. Do not attempt any vigorous stretching, although gentle mobilisation of the joints is essential to prevent even more loss of movement and stiffness. I have numerous patients who would not give up their precious treatments for anything.

Older people derive great pleasure from having their hands and feet massaged and these areas are readily accessible. Great comfort and pain relief can result from stretching the fingers and toes and mobilising the joints. Bend and stretch all the joints and move ankles and wrists in a circular motion to improve the range of movement. Treatment of the hands and feet is a good introduction to massage and the receiver may decide to disrobe fully and enjoy an all-over massage.

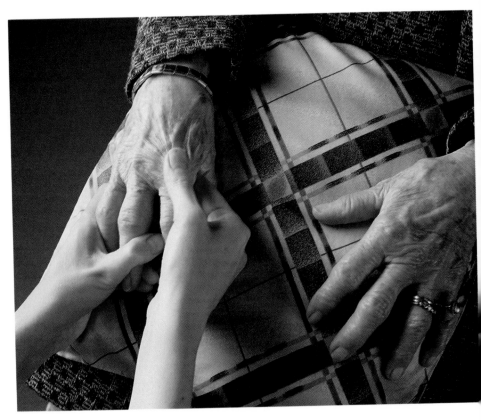

Essential oils which are beneficial for arthritis include: **chamomile**, **cypress**, **eucalyptus**, **lavender**, **lemon**, **peppermint** and **rosemary**.

Since arthritis and other ailments can begin in the mind the Bach Flower Remedies may prove to be of immense value. If the thoughts are positive then the problem will often be alleviated or may even disappear. The following remedies may be indicated in later life:

Gorse

- For hopelessness and despair when you are at the 'end of the road' when you are suffering from chronic disease.

Heather

- For constantly dwelling on personal problems. Many in this state are completely self-obsessed and will tell their entire medical history to anyone, even a stranger.

Honeysuckle

- For clinging to the past. This is an excellent remedy for bereavement.

Mustard

- For depression which apparently has no specific cause.

Olive

- For tiredness and exhaustion.

Pine

- For guilt.

Rock rose

- For panic attacks, phobias (e.g. agoraphobia).

Vine

- For rigid attitude and domineering tendencies.

Walnut

- For change e.g. retirement, bereavement, terminal illness.

Willow

- For bitterness and resentment.

General aches and sprains

Massage can play a major role in the alleviation of all aches and pains wherever they may be. Fresh blood is brought to the affected muscles and any toxins which have accumulated are removed. Most people will suffer at some time in their life from aches caused by stress, bad posture, gardening, sport and so on. Useful essential oils include: **chamomile**, **eucalyptus**, **lavender**, **lemon**, **peppermint** and **rosemary**.

Sprains

The ankle is the most commonly sprained joint and will be swollen and hot with extreme pain on movement. An ice pack should be applied immediately. If you do not have one then improvise by wrapping a tea-towel around a packet of frozen peas! Cold compresses are also useful for reducing inflammation and heat whilst easing the pain. Follow the compress with a massage blend taking care not to massage *directly* onto the affected joint. Useful oils include **chamomile**, **eucalyptus**, **lavender**, **peppermint** and **rosemary**.

Respiratory problems

All respiratory problems from simple coughs and colds to chronic bronchial conditions will improve with regular use of massage. The state of deep relaxation which occurs as a result of the treatment allows the breathing to slow down and deepen. This is important since emotional factors and stress always worsen bronchial problems. It is particularly important to concentrate on the thoracic area of the back. The percussion movements, cupping and hacking, stimulate the respiratory system and encourage the removal of mucus.

Those with respiratory problems such as asthma and bronchitis do not usually breathe properly and engage in shallow chest breathing. They gasp their way through life forcing themselves to survive on shallower and shallower breaths. Breathing takes place totally in the chest, and the lower portion of the lungs which should be supplying 80 per cent of the oxygen to the body is never utilised.

Deep abdominal breathing exercises should be practised daily by those with chronic problems. In fact the benefits are marvellous for everyone and we should all practise deep abdominal breathing. Stress is relieved immediately, relaxation induced and pressure is taken off the heart.

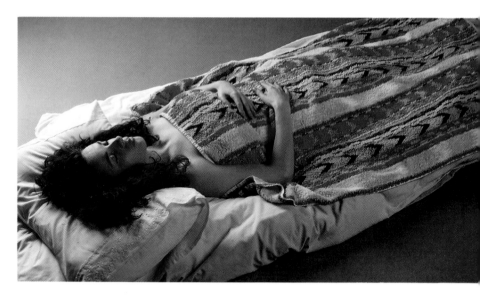

Either sit up or lie down. Place one hand below the navel and one hand above it. As you breathe in for six counts feel the abdomen fill with air and then hold the breath for two counts. Now breathe out for six counts – the hand positioned above the navel will move prior to the lower hand. Breathe like this for approximately five minutes daily and you will notice a remarkable difference.

It is also highly recommended to open a window at night whilst sleeping. Every time you exhale, the levels of carbon dioxide and other

poisons increase in your bedroom and you will start to breathe them back
in again unless there is a supply of fresh air.

Diet is obviously a contributory factor. By avoiding in particular, dairy
foods and sugar and trying not to combine proteins and carbohydrates
together at the same meal, vast improvements can be made. Dairy foods,
in particular, encourage the production of mucus. It is a misconception
that we need these foods. Readily absorbable calcium may be obtained
from green leafy vegetables and raw nuts.

Remember that essential oils added to the carrier oil will increase the
effectiveness of the massage. You may also decide to purchase a small
clay burner. Put a few teaspoons of water into the loose bowl on the top
and sprinkle approximately 6 drops of essential oil into it (see the list of
suggested oils below). Light the nightlight to diffuse the oils.
Alternatively simply place 6 drops of your chosen oil into any small bowl
of water and place the bowl in a warm place. To prevent the spread of
infection when someone in your household has a cold use a small plant
spray filled with water to which you have added approximately 10 drops
of essential oil.

The following oils from our Top 10 will be helpful:

Asthma and bronchitis

- Cypress, eucalyptus, lavender, lemon, peppermint and rosemary.

Breath (shortness of)

- Lavender.

Catarrh

- Eucalyptus, lavender, lemon and rosemary.

Coughs/colds/flu

- Eucalyptus, lavender, lemon, peppermint, rosemary and sandalwood.

Sinusitis

- Eucalyptus, lavender.

Spasmodic coughs

- Cypress.

Throat infections

- Eucalyptus, geranium, lavender, lemon and sandalwood.

During asthma attacks the Bach Flower Rescue Remedy is indispensable
for calming the person. Where extreme terror and fear or sheer panic
are present then **rock rose** should be administered. **Olive** is excellent for
the ensuing exhaustion after an attack. Take **mimulus** where there is fear
of future asthma attacks since fear will often attract the very thing you
are afraid of.

Neurological/emotional problems

Headache or migraine

Virtually all headaches originate from tension in the neck and shoulders. Regular neck massage, paying particular attention to the base of the skull, will reduce the number of headaches occurring and may even eradicate them completely. Facial/scalp massage is also indicated. Spend extra time on the forehead, where many people carry a great deal of their tension, and also to the jaw line, since anxious individuals often grind their teeth at night. Essential oils for headaches include: **chamomile** (calming and soothing, pain relieving), **lavender** (calming, pain relieving, sedative) and **peppermint** (pain relieving, cooling).

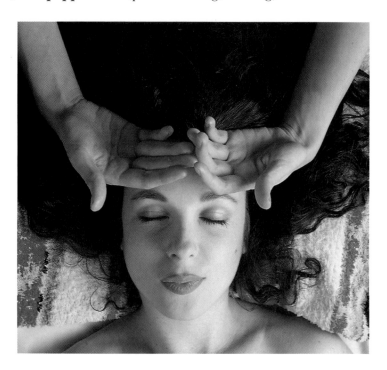

Where migraine is prevalent it can have many causes. It is often due to living in the 'fast lane' when the sudden relaxation at weekends brings on an attack. Many sufferers are allergic to certain foods and should try cutting out those commonly linked with migraine, such as cheese, coffee, chocolate and red wine. Stress, of course, is also a major contributory cause.

In my years as a therapist I have encountered many desperate migraine patients who had tried every therapy without effect and I was their last hope. They have been amazed by the benefits afforded by massage.

When the head is too sensitive to be massaged in the midst of a migraine attack, put two drops of pure essential oil of **lavender** onto a finger and very gently dab it onto the forehead and temples. You may also sprinkle one drop of **lavender** and one drop of **chamomile** onto a tissue and inhale deeply. It is important to use oils at the onset of an attack to eradicate the migraine completely.

Since headaches may be caused by too much worrying, the Bach Flower Remedies may be required. **Red chestnut** is indicated for excessive anxiety and concern for the safety of others e.g. thinking an accident has occurred because someone is five minutes late. Those who require **white chestnut** suffer from unwanted thoughts that go round and round in the head all day and all night long. They are unable to sleep, tired, depressed and full of stress. No wonder they suffer from headaches!

Insomnia

Almost all of us suffer from insomnia at sometime during our lives. It is usually stress-related but can also have other causes, such as eating too late before retiring. If sleepless nights are a problem then try to avoid all stimulating drinks such as tea and coffee before bedtime. Replace these drinks with a herb tea. Insomnia is a habit which needs to be broken.

Regular weekly massage will ease insomnia. Try massaging your own neck, shoulders and face every evening (see Chapter 9). To encourage sleep try **chamomile**, **lavender**, **sandalwood** and **ylang ylang**. You may wish to sprinkle one drop of **chamomile** and one drop of **lavender** onto your pillow.

Skin problems

The skin is prone to many disorders. It often reflects the inner state of health of the individual and sometimes is the first part of the body to manifest disease occurring elsewhere.

Acne

Acne particularly strikes teenagers and although it is only a minor disorder it can be very disfiguring and creates much depression and anxiety in younger people. The basic cause may be an over-production of sebum which clogs up the pores, resulting in blackheads and whiteheads. Diet is also a contributory factor and it is important to eat a healthy, balanced diet containing mostly fruit and vegetables and avoiding sugar, refined and fatty foods. Stress can also result in the over-production of sebum.

Massage the face daily adding **chamomile**, **geranium**, **lavender**, or **lemon** to your carrier oil.

Eczema

Eczema is not infectious and is generally due to an allergic reaction to any of a large number of substances such as dairy foods, wheat, cosmetics and household detergents. Emotional problems may also cause an outbreak of eczema. It is a matter of finding the cause and eliminating it. Useful oils are **chamomile** (due to its anti-inflammatory and anti-allergic properties), **geranium** and **lavender** (for their balancing and healing qualities) and **sandalwood** (for dry skin).

Athlete's foot

The warm, damp conditions in training shoes provide the perfect environment for this fungal infection to develop. Wash the feet daily, drying them thoroughly and afterwards massage with any vegetable oil to which you have added **lavender** and **lemon**. You may also apply a couple of drops of neat essential oil to the infected toes.

Chilblains

Chilblains are due to poor circulation and regular massage will undoubtedly improve this condition. Daily exercise is also advisable to reduce the occurrence of chilblains. Essential oils of **geranium** and **lemon** may be helpful to add to your carrier oil.

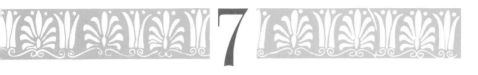

7

MASSAGE FOR PREGNANCY AND CHILDBIRTH

Pregnancy

During pregnancy a woman undergoes enormous physical and emotional changes. Massage provides an extremely safe and gentle alternative to drugs for the many minor ailments that may occur. Obviously medical intervention is sometimes necessary, but massage will help to promote a very healthy and happy pregnancy. I have massaged many women throughout their pregnancy and I have only ever received positive reactions. They have enjoyed a much improved sleep pattern, backache and muscle cramps have been considerably reduced, headaches and constipation have been relieved, indigestion and heartburn have been minimal and tension, depression and mood swings have been alleviated. Varicose veins in the legs, caused by all the added pressure of the baby, have been avoided due to the improvements in circulation. A pregnant woman should always be encouraged to listen to her body – if she feels tired then she must rest.

Throughout pregnancy, especially for the first three months, your movements should be very gentle. When massaging the lower back and abdomen take special care. Do not use deep pressure or percussion movements.

Take great care using essential oils as some are contraindicated during pregnancy due to the danger of miscarriage. The safest and most useful oils to choose are **lavender** and **tangerine**.

Back massage

A pregnant woman will obviously find it uncomfortable to lie on her front. She can either sit astride a chair with a cushion between her abdomen and the chair back or she may prefer to adopt a side-lying position.

Kneel behind her using a cushion under your own knees. Commence at the bottom of her back and using effleurage movements proceed up towards the top of the back and up and around the shoulders and glide back down to your starting point applying no pressure.

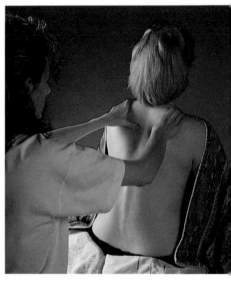

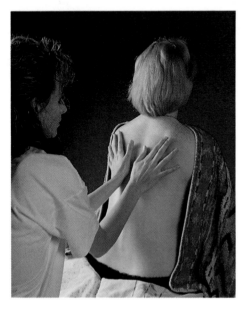

The kneading movements of picking up and rolling and wringing may be applied to the top of the shoulders. Finish with more stroking effleurage movements.

You may then perform the small circular friction movements either side of the spine but apply only *gentle* pressure. Repeat the effleurage. Use circular friction movements around both the shoulder blades to alleviate tension – firmer pressure may be employed.

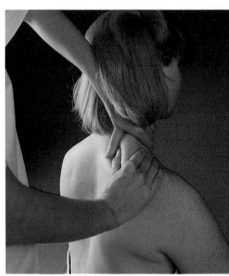

Leg massage

Massage to the legs is great for improving circulation, alleviating fluid retention and cramp and for preventing varicose veins. The pregnant woman should adopt a side-lying position and lots of gentle stroking effleurage movements can be applied. Follow my routine for leg massage but omit the percussion movements.

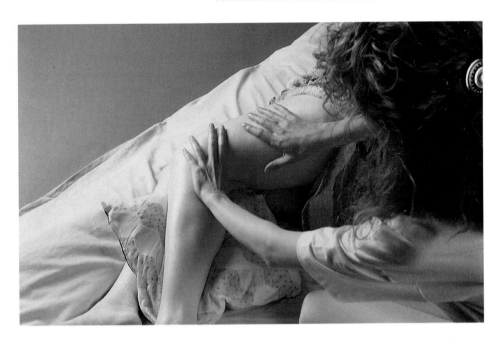

Front of the body

Whilst treating the front of the body use plenty of cushions under the head and shoulders and under the knees to relieve pressure on the lower back.

Abdominal massage

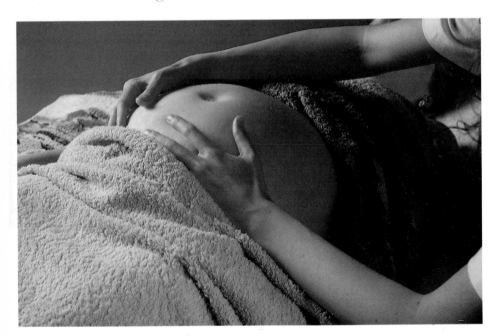

Apply very gentle effleurage movements ensuring that you are proceeding in a clockwise direction. Do **not** perform the kidney drainage or percussion movements. Colon massage should be very light.

Abdominal massage is marvellous for constipation, easing indigestion, helping to prevent stretchmarks and relieving taut, stretched skin. Pregnant mothers can also massage themselves to establish early bonding and to calm down an active baby at night-time!

Breast massage

Breasts may become tender, especially at the beginning of pregnancy. Soreness can be minimised by gently stroking the breasts in a circular direction towards the armpits.

Facial massage

An excellent method of relieving the stresses and strains of pregnancy. Follow my sequence already described to eradicate headaches and to induce calmness and reassurance. Most pregnant women love facial massage!

Childbirth

Massage is invaluable at this time. It is an effective way to reduce low back pain, to help regulate contractions and to speed up the delivery. It also provides the comfort and support which a labouring woman so badly needs. You must be very patient as some pregnant women do not like to be touched when in labour.

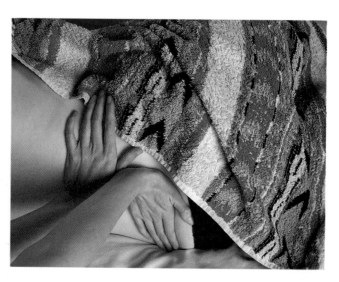

Use lower back massage with the receiver in a side-lying position. Very deep pressure is required to afford pain relief. Foot massage is also desirable during childbirth. Cold **lavender** compresses may be placed on the forehead to calm the woman or on the lower back and abdomen to reduce pain.

Bach Flower Remedies

The Bach Flower Remedies are extremely useful for pregnant women both in the pre- and post-natal periods when mood swings are so prevalent. It is vital that these are balanced since a happy pregnant woman will usually have a far easier labour and delivery and a more contented baby. **Schleranthus** will aid these extreme fluctuations of mood and instability. Two of the most useful remedies in pregnancy are **Rescue Remedy** for apprehension and **walnut** for the profound changes which are occurring. I highly recommend that **Rescue Remedy** be administered two weeks before the due date, four times a day. It will relax the mother dispelling fear and panic to ensure a speedier and less painful delivery and a faster recovery. As the big day approaches, **mimulus** may also be required for fear and apprehension. Extreme fear demands **rock rose**. During the delivery **vervain** and **impatiens** may be employed along with **Rescue Remedy** to calm the mind and relax the body. After the birth I highly recommend **olive**. This helps to alleviate the exhaustion felt by the mother.

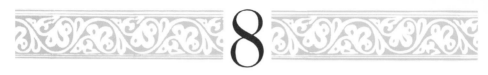

8

MASSAGE FOR BABIES

The first sense developed by the embryo is that of touch as it is rocked and nourished in the mother's womb, constantly embraced in amniotic fluid. Babies need the familiar sensation of constant reassuring and loving touch after they enter the world. Massage will help to create a very close and loving bond between mother, father and baby. It assists in both the physiological and the emotional development of the child. Evidence suggests that babies receiving massage experience far fewer health problems. I have two children, one of three years and the other one year old and fortunately they have never required a doctor's attention.

Digestion and elimination is improved, with babies suffering far less from colic, constipation and diarrhoea. The nervous system is calmed, resulting in less irritability and easier nights for the parents. The respiratory system is also assisted, resulting in fewer coughs, colds, nasal and ear infections. The baby's joints and muscles become far more flexible and supple. Baby massage should help your child to become a well-balanced individual later on in life. To massage a baby is also beneficial to the parents as it lowers stress levels and restores calmness and tranquillity.

When and where to massage

Always be responsive to the mood of your baby. It is pointless to attempt a massage when the baby is hungry, restless, irritable or overtired. Usually about half-an-hour after a feed is an appropriate time. Babies have a short attention span and are easily tired so it is advisable to establish a regular massage routine – for instance before a night-time bath. Ten minutes will probably be sufficient. Always ensure that the room is very warm since babies lose heat so quickly.

Pressure should be light and gentle and almost like a game. Do not adhere rigidly to my suggested routine. Follow your own intuition for you and the baby will know what is best. When massaging either sit back comfortably supported against some cushions with knees bent and the baby resting on your thighs or place the baby on the floor on a nice thick duvet covered with a warm soft towel.

Use a light vegetable oil easily absorbed by the skin, such as sweet almond or grapeseed oil. Baby oil is not a suitable medium as it does not penetrate satisfactorily. Take great care with essential oils. I advise the use of one drop of **lavender** or **Roman chamomile**. Only add one drop of essential oil to about 15 ml (one tablespoonful) of carrier oil.

Suggested routine

As I have already stated, just do what feels natural and if the baby becomes bored do not persevere, try later. Perform each movement about three to four times.

It is a good idea to commence on the front of the body as this will make the baby feel secure as he or she can see your face.

Legs

A baby is fascinated by the toes and will love to watch you as you massage. Hold your baby's foot and stroke the leg from thigh to ankle. Stroke the foot and rotate the ankle gently and then stretch and rotate each toe. Bend and stretch the knee slowly. Now repeat on the other side.

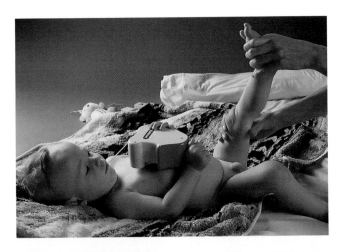

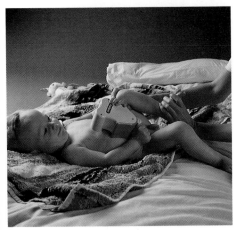

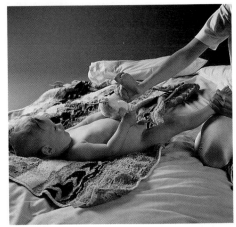

Abdomen and shoulders

With both hands stroke up the front of the body and over the shoulders and let both hands glide back.

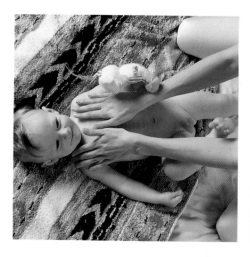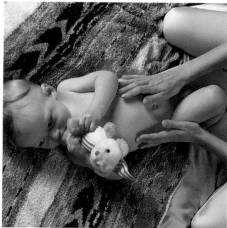

Place one hand on top of the other on the abdomen and with featherlight touch move in a clockwise direction. This is marvellous for stomach aches!

Place both hands on the baby's breast bone and lightly stroke hands across the top of the chest.

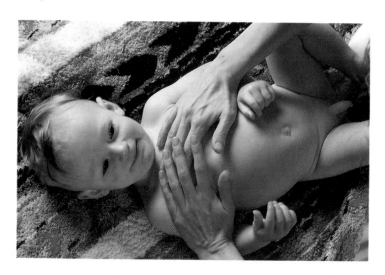

Arms

Hold the baby's hand and stroke the arm from the fingers to the shoulder. Rotate the wrist and then stretch and circle each finger slowly.

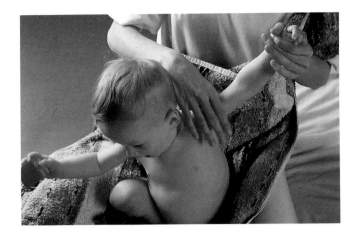

Bend both the baby's elbows and then take both arms out to the side and across the chest and up and over the top of the head and down again.

Face

Stroke gently from the top of the head down the sides of the face to the chin.

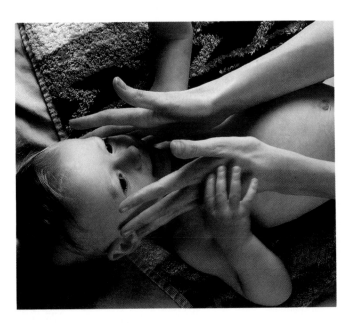

Stroke across the forehead, across the cheeks and across the chin. Make circles around the eye area with the index finger and also around the mouth.

To connect the front of the body stroke your hands from the top of the head, down the chest and abdomen and down the legs.

Back of the body

Stroke from the ankles up the legs right over the buttocks, up the back and then return to your starting position with absolutely no pressure. Stroke each buttock using a circular movement and then gently squeeze each buttock.

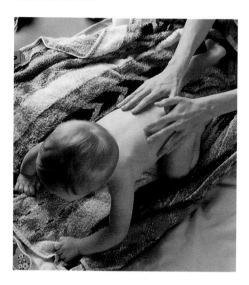

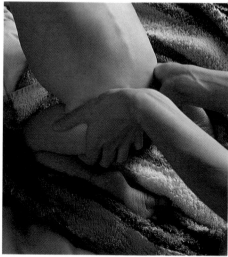

Place one hand either side of the spine so that they look like the wings of a bird and stroke each hand gently outwards.

To connect the back of the body glide both hands from baby's head down to the feet. Finish with a cuddle!

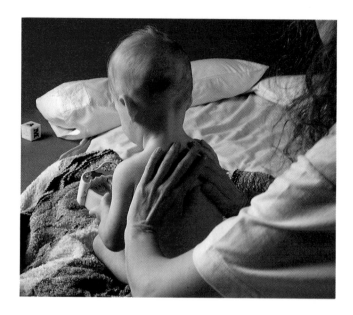

Bach Flower Remedies for babies

Since the Bach Flower Remedies carry no side-effects they can be used very safely on babies and children who will respond very quickly. I have found the following remedies of great benefit:

Chicory

- Most children need this! For a restless clinging baby who constantly seeks attention and does not like to be alone.

Clematis

- For a sleepy drowsy baby who apparently takes no interest in anything. This baby will not even bother to wake up for a feed.

Mimulus

- To be prescribed for very nervous and fearful babies. They will always cry on awakening. An older child may be given this for his/her known fears e.g. fear of the dark.

Impatiens

- Impatient, quick tempered babies (and parents!) require this.

Star of Bethlehem

- A useful remedy for the shock and trauma of the birth, particularly when there has been some difficulty.

Vervain

- For the over-active baby who will not sleep.

Dosage

- If the mother is breast feeding she should take the remedies herself and the benefit will be imparted to the infant through her milk two feeds later. If the child is bottle fed then the usual four drops should be added to the bottle of milk four times daily.

9

SELF-MASSAGE

Obviously there are several disadvantages to self-massage. There are some areas of the body which you cannot reach without stretching and other areas which you cannot reach with dexterity and force. Also you cannot relax totally since one part of your body is obliged to massage. In addition no transmission of energy takes place from one person to another.

However, self-massage does have advantages. It is an excellent method of discovering what feels good and does not feel good. It is an invaluable tool to use for feedback purposes. It will teach you a great deal about your body and the more you know about how to massage your own body the more capable you will be to deal with others' bodies. You know more than anyone else where it really hurts. You will be able to soothe away your own aches and pains whenever you wish.

Legs

Leg massage will relieve the aches and pains of the day when you have been standing or sitting for long periods of time and will relieve the tiredness of over-exercised muscles.

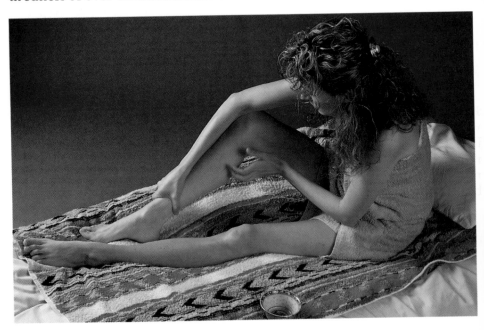

Sit down on the floor with your legs outstretched in front of you. Stroke the entire leg from ankle to thigh so that the lymph is encouraged to flow towards the lymph glands in the groin. Bend the knee so that you can friction around the ankle joint to loosen it. Keep the knee bent to work on the foot. Friction the sole of the foot. Stretch each toe individually and circle them in both directions.

You may find it easier to massage the foot if you rest one foot on the opposite thigh. You may need to rest your bent knee on a cushion.

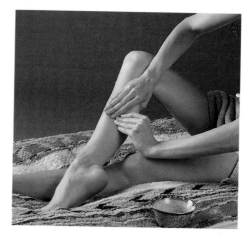

knee with the circular friction movements. Moving up to the thigh, perform kneading movements on the front, inside

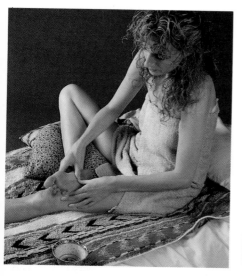

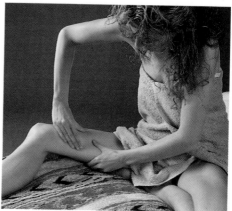

Keep the knee bent so that you can work on the calf muscles at the back of the leg. Use kneading movements for this area and then massage the lymph nodes at the back of the knee. Work around the

and outside of the thigh. Regular kneading of the calf muscles can improve the shape and tone and can help to reduce cellulite on the thighs. Finish with an effleurage of the whole leg.

Hips and buttocks

Work deeply all over the hip and buttock area using squeezing kneading movements. Make a fist and try a pummelling action to break down the fatty tissue. Roll onto your other side and repeat.

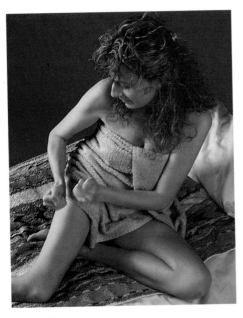

Abdomen

Lying on your back with your legs bent up to ensure relaxation of the abdominal area work in a clockwise direction employing the stroking

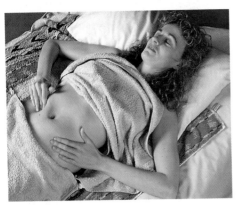

effleurage action. Start at the bottom right-hand side of the abdomen performing gentle friction movements working in the direction of the colon – i.e. bottom right-hand side to top right-hand side, to top left-hand side and down to lower left-hand side. This is an excellent way to relieve constipation and gripy pains. Some gentle cupping may be executed to enhance and stimulate digestion.

Neck and shoulders

The simplest way to massage these areas is sitting on a chair or the floor but you may lie on your back if you wish. Sitting in the chair let your head hang forward and pressing as hard as you can with the fingertips make the small circular friction movements at the base of the skull.

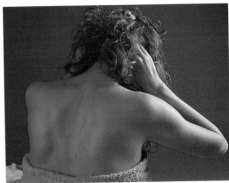

Bring your head upright and squeeze the left shoulder by reaching across the front of the body with the right hand.

Repeat on the right shoulder using the left hand. If you are able to reach across the back of the body then press as hard as you can working across the top of the shoulder blade towards the spine.

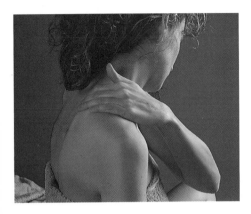

Try to work a little way down the shoulder blade too.

Back

Obviously this is a difficult area to reach but we all suffer from aches and pains in the lower back so it is worth persevering. Either standing up or sitting down press the tips of your thumbs as hard as possible into the dimples on either side of the spine. Work up the spine as hard as you can.

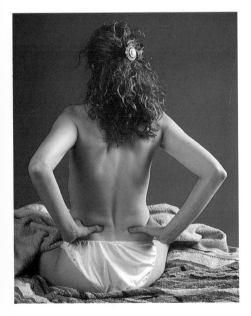

Arms and hands

Lying down or sitting up, effleurage each arm working from the wrist up to the shoulder endeavouring to move the lymph into the armpit region. Work the hands. Stretch, flex and extend and circle the fingers and move the wrists from side to side and round and round. Firmly effleurage the lower arm and then bend and stretch the elbow as far as you can. Wring the upper arm. Work around the front and back of the shoulder joint. Repeat on the other arm. Finally reach both arms over your head and really stretch.

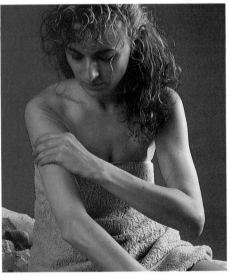

Face and scalp

Lie down on your back to increase relaxation. Using the fingertips rub the scalp vigorously all over in a circular motion. Stroke the forehead with the fingertips working from the centre out towards the hairline. Make circular movements with the fingers all over the ears and pull them gently.

Run your fingers through the hair.
Place both hands on the temples to
finish and relax.

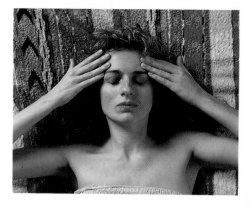

Massage is such a wonderful way to relax completely, unwind and
revitalise, and I guarantee that it will add a whole new dimension to your
life. You will wonder how you ever managed to survive before without
the magical language of touch. Try to swap a massage every week with a
friend. It is just as important to care for yourself as it is to care for others!

FURTHER READING

Bek L. and Pullar P., *The Seven Levels of Healing*, Rider, London, 1986
Bek L. and Pullar., *To the Light*, Unwin, London, 1986
Brown D., *Headway Lifeguides: Aromatherapy*, Hodder & Stoughton, Sevenoaks, 1993
Chancellor P.M., *Illustrated Handbook of the Bach Flower Remedies*, C.W. Daniel, 1971
Diamond H. and M., *Fit for Life*, Bantum Press, London, 1987
Grant D. and Joice J., *Food Combining for Health*, Thorsons, London, 1984
Kenton L. and S., *Raw Energy*, Century, London, 1984
Valnet Dr J., *The Practice of Aromatherapy*, C.W. Daniel, 1982
Walker Dr N.W., *Diet and Salad*, Norwalk Press, 1971

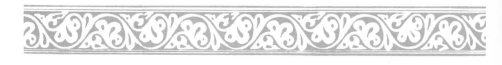

USEFUL ADDRESSES

Beaumont College of Natural Medicine
16 Dittons Road
Eastbourne
East Sussex BN21 1DW
Tel: 0323 724855/641676

For information on professional training courses under the direction of Denise Brown, pure essential oils, base oils, music cassettes, videos, etc.

British and European Osteopathic Association
6 Adelaide Road
Teddington
Middlesex TW11 0AY
Tel: 081 977 8532

The U.K. Homoeopathic Medicine Association
243, The Broadway
Southall
Middlesex UB1 1NF

The Society of Homoeopaths
2 Artisan Road
Northampton NN1 4HU
Tel: 0604 21400

I.S.P.A. (International Society of Professional Aromatherapists)
41 Leicester Road
Hinckley
Leicestershire LE10 1LW
Tel: 0455 637687

For a list of fully qualified therapists in your area.

I.F.A. (International Federation of Aromatherapy)
Department of Continuing Education
The Royal Masonic Hospital
Ravenscourt Park
London W6 0TW
Tel: 081 846 8066

For a list of fully qualified therapists in your area

Aromatherapy Organisation Council
3 Latymer Close
Braybrooke
Market Harborough
Leicestershire LE16 8LN

Natural Hygiene Society
Dr K. Sidhwa
3 Harold Grove
Frinton-on-Sea
Essex

The Cranial Osteopathic Association
478 Baker Street
Enfield
Middlesex EN1 3QS
Tel: 081 367 5561